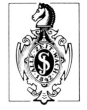

John Dobbing (Ed.)

A Balanced Diet?

With 29 Figures

Springer-Verlag
London Berlin Heidelberg New York
Paris Tokyo

John Dobbing, DSc, FRCP, FRCPath
Emeritus Professor of Child Growth and Development, Department of
Child Health, University of Manchester, Oxford Road,
Manchester M13 9PT, UK

ISBN 3–540–19527–0   Springer-Verlag Berlin Heidelberg New York
ISBN 0–387–19527–0   Springer-Verlag New York Berlin Heidelberg

British Library Cataloguing in Publication Data
A balanced diet?
1. Man. Health. Effects of diet
I. Dobbing, John, *1922–*
613.2
ISBN 3–540–19527–0

Library of Congress Cataloging-in-Publication Data
A Balanced diet? / [edited by] John Dobbing.
p.   cm.
Bibliography: p.   Includes index.
ISBN 0–387–19527–0 (US)
1. Nutritionally induced diseases 2. Nutrition. I. Dobbing, John.
RC622.B35 1988 616.3′9—dc19

© Springer-Verlag Berlin Heidelberg 1988

Printed in Great Britain

Filmset by Tradeset, Welwyn Garden City, Herts
Printed by Henry Ling, The Dorset Press, Dorchester

2128/3830-543210

Preface

Most multi-author books are either "books of scientific meetings" or collections of essays written by people selected by the Editor and invited to write around a common subject. This one is of neither type. It is the eighth in a series of "Dobbing Workshops" which began as an experiment in 1980, designed to avoid some of the disadvantages of both.

By far the greatest disadvantage of most orthodox multi-author books is that, unlike the papers in normal scientific research journals, they are not subjected to the usual refereeing procedure known as "peer review". They are too frequently a means of by which authors can perpetrate, unchallenged, the publication of their own personal views, idiosyncrasies and straight mistakes in archival form. This should never happen, and only rarely does so, in the standard research journals, in which the reader can at least be assured that someone, usually far more knowledgeable than he, has had the opportunity to criticise the manuscript. What he reads is to that limited extent not likely to be flagrant rubbish. Such a time-honoured system does not, of course, guarantee complete probity, but at least the literature is less cluttered than it otherwise would be by wrong, misleading or trivial material. Peer review is not, however, without its own problems, since the chosen peer, being usually an acknowledged expert, and therefore a pillar of the Establishment, may frown on genuine innovation, as well as the rubbish, thereby inhibiting progress. Nevertheless it is a better system than the unreviewed publication in which everyone is his own expert, and much can be done to avoid unfair judgement by appointing more than one peer to comment on a submitted paper – this being the usual procedure. Would that lay authors, including journalists, often espousing activist causes, were subject to a similar discipline! There would then be less dangerously misleading writing, and much less flatulence from an increasing number who presently pervert the cause of consumerism for their own gratification.

Our new system goes some way towards avoiding some of these difficulties by having all the contributors to the book extensively referee all of the chapters.

On this occasion the contributors were chosen by Professor Donald Naismith, an established nutritionist, who contributed the first chapter and submitted like everyone else to the peer review system to be outlined.

Each author's paper was first sent to all the other authors, who were asked to write a critical commentary on it as though they were doing so for a scientific journal – a procedure with which, as practising scientists, they were all familiar. All the critical commentaries were then sent to all the authors. At this stage an author could react to criticism in one of three ways: he could modify his original manuscript to take account of the criticism; or he could write a reply, to be published alongside the commentary; or he could ignore the criticism altogether.

We then all met for three days as a committee, and worked through each chapter in turn and thrashed out persisting disagreements. Sometimes during our meetings new topics or new points on existing topics arose, and someone would be asked to write a new paragraph or so for publication in the commentary. The finished book therefore contains a series of chapters, extensively peer reviewed like few others, followed by a "scrapbook" of residual commentary. There was absolutely no intention to reach a consensus on any matter. Consensus at the frontiers of scientific thought and knowledge spells death to progress, and dullness in the form of a lowest common denominator.

The main way our system differed from the reviewing practices of the learned scientific journal was that the sole judge of what was ultimately published was the author himself. Both in the chapters and the commentary which follows them, the named author has been exclusively responsible for what appears; but each has had the advantage of knowing precisely what eight other experts thought of his contribution. All the contributors know the extent to which their original writings were modified in the light of such refining fire. You, as the reader, will not be able to detect this, but at least you will be reassured that the quality of what you read has been enhanced, without detracting from the author's own views and style.

Such an exercise costs money, though not a very great deal. For generously agreeing to provide this, we wish to express our gratitude to the Snack, Nut and Crisps Manufacturers' Association. Since it has regrettably become customary to be suspicious that the sponsor may in some way have manipulated the occasion to his own advantage, I can only say that I am not aware of this having happened in this case. Part of my own role as Editor and Chairman was to act as honest broker, and to intervene and protect, where necessary, the interests of the participants from the sponsor. I can only say that such was never necessary. Furthermore, for the activist or the sceptic, I would like to hear of any part of the book which directly favours SNACMA in betrayal of the scientific truth. I have not found one. To be sure, such sponsorship is rarely altruistic, since a sponsor gains by being known, as in this case, to be prepared to take an important public and scientific topic seriously. Far from begrudging them that, I am profoundly grateful.

I wish to thank Keith Nightingale of SNACMA for a quality of helpfulness and personal kindness and tolerance which is rare; and my wife, Dr. Jean Sands, for almost comparable tolerance, but above all for her expert scientific and secretarial help. Finally I owe much to all the contributors, who have had to put up with my substantial importunities, especially in the run-up period.

Hayfield, January 1988   John Dobbing

Contents

Contributors

M. E. J. Curzon, BDS, PhD, LDSRCS, FRCD(C)
Professor of Child Dental Health and Preventive Dentistry, University
of Leeds, Woodhouse Lane, Leeds LS2 9JT

John Dobbing, DSc, FRCP, FRCPath (Editor and Chairman)
Emeritus Professor of Child Growth and Development, University of
Manchester, Oxford Road, Manchester M13 9PT

J. V. G. A. Durnin, MA, DSc, FRCP, FRSE
Institute of Physiology, University of Glasgow, Glasgow G12 8QQ

R. J. Jarrett, MA, MD, FFCM
Professor of Clinical Epidemiology, United Medical and Dental Schools
of Guy's and St. Thomas's Hospitals, University of London, Guy's
Campus, London SE1 9RT

I. Macdonald MD, DSc, FIBiol
Professor of Physiology, United Medical and Dental Schools of Guy's
and St. Thomas's Hospitals, University of London, Guy's Campus,
London SE1 9RT

G. A. MacGregor, FRCP
Senior Lecturer and Honorary Consultant Physician, Blood Pressure
Unit, Department of Medicine, Charing Cross and Westminster Medical
School, University of London, The Reynolds Building, St. Dunstan's
Road, London W6 8RP

D. J. Naismith, PhD
Professor of Nutrition, Department of Food and Nutritional Sciences,
King's College London, Campden Hill Road, London W8 7AH

J. P. W. Rivers, BSc, MIBiol
Senior Lecturer, Department of Human Nutrition, London School of
Hygiene and Tropical Medicine, University of London, Keppel Street,
London W1

T. A. B. Sanders, PhD
Lecturer in Nutrition, Department of Food and Nutritional Sciences,
King's College London, Campden Hill Road, London W8 7AH

D. A. T. Southgate, PhD
Head of Nutrition and Food Quality Department, AFRC Institute of
Food Research, Colney Lane, Norwich NR4 7UA

J. E. Thomas, BSc, MMedSci, SRD
Lecturer, Department of Food and Nutritional Sciences, King's College
London, Campden Hill Road, London W8 7AH

Chapter 1

Diet and Health: Striking a Balance

D. J. Naismith

It has recently been suggested [1] that the term "a balanced diet" is outdated, having served its purpose in contributing to the eradication of deficiency diseases, and should be replaced by another which embodies a more explicit reference to the role of diet in the development of the chronic degenerative diseases that afflict all industrialised countries, and the affluent subgroups in Third World populations. Terms such as "the prudent diet" and "the healthful diet" have gained some ground in the United States, but they in turn would have to be explained.

Following the identification of the nutrients, and elucidation of their physiological properties – a process that is by no means complete – the concept of an ideal balance within the diet emerged. This has been the cornerstone of all nutrition education programmes, and of nutrition planning at all levels, from the provision of school meals to the modulation of agricultural policies.

A balanced diet has several essential features. It must satisfy minimum physiological needs for all the nutrients and energy, in order to avoid clinically manifest deficiencies. This aspect has tended to dominate nutrition thinking in traditional health education, although it is largely irrelevant in contemporary Britain. Since nutrient and energy requirements change with age, with physiological status and with lifestyle, it follows that the proportions of nutrients within the balanced diet and their relationship to total energy intake must also change. Thus there is no one optimal diet for all groups within the population. However, since most diets consumed in economically prosperous countries invariably provide protein, fat, vitamins and minerals in considerable excess then factors other than satisfying physiological needs may be of greater significance.

The most important are the possible risks to health arising from overconsumption of certain nutrients and foods such as fat, protein, the fat-soluble vitamins and sugar, and the effect of one dietary component consumed in excess on the utilisation of others. For example, dietary fibre, which is believed to have many beneficial properties, is known to interfere with the absorption of trace elements. In addition to preventing nutrient deficiency, a balanced diet should have a composition that is compatible with the maintenance of optimal health throughout life.

It is often claimed by health educators that a balanced diet can be achieved by as varied a selection of foods as possible. There is no doubt that the lack of variety in the diets of most people in developing countries, especially those dependent on one staple food for the provision of the bulk of dietary energy, may be a factor often associated with such classical deficiency diseases as xerophthalmia, pellagra and beriberi. The great diversity of fresh and processed foods to be found in any modern supermarket, which has eliminated the influences of regional production (apart from peculiar regional preferences) and seasonal availability, has not, however, guaranteed that nutritional deficiencies are no longer seen, or that a healthy diet is enjoyed by all. Indeed many believe that the increasing use of convenience foods, processed foods and snack foods, which feature prominently in the modern diet, and particularly so in that of young teenagers, is the principal cause of the so-called diseases of affluence.

The term "balance" refers to the ultimate proportions of the nutrients resulting from combining different foods; the composition of individual foods (fresh fruit, snack foods, confectionery) is important only in the context of the extent to which they contribute to the total food energy. Since intakes of the nutrients vary very considerably from day to day, the idea of a balanced food, or even a balanced meal, has little meaning. Balance is achieved over a period of days.

Meeting Physiological Needs

In the population of the United Kingdom, as in most industrialised countries, nutritional deficiency diseases no longer constitute a significant public health problem. Nutrient needs are satisfied in the great majority. It is important to distinguish between nutrient deficiency diseases and low intakes of the nutrients. These are often confused, and individuals with poor nutritional status, as revealed by measurements of food consumption or the analysis of blood, are often described as being "deficient", although clinical signs of deficiency are rarely seen.

The advantage of most biochemical tests is that they reveal "subclinical" deficiency, i.e. a potential functional impairment. A man with a haemoglobin concentration of 12 g/100 ml blood would be described as anaemic according to the conventional (arbitrary) definition [2], yet Davies et al. [3] found significant changes in physical performance only when the haemoglobin concentration fell below 10 g/100 ml. To give further examples, the tryptophan load test is used to challenge a metabolic pathway regulated by a pyridoxine-dependent enzyme, and thus to detect subclinical pyridoxine deficiency. Clinical deficiency of this vitamin is, however, extremely rare, and the load employed (2 g tryptophan) is equivalent to the consumption, at one meal, of one and a half pounds (681 g) of lean beef. A low leucocyte concentration of ascorbic acid is not accompanied by clinical symptoms of scurvy, or even ill-health in the subject. All of these biochemical measurements are useful in identifying suboptimal intakes of nutrients (i.e. below the Recommended Daily Allowance, or RDA) that dietary measurements could not establish with certainty.

Within any population a wide range of intakes, particularly of the micronutrients (vitamins and minerals, including the trace elements), is usually found, and a small proportion with intakes at the lower end of the range may ultimately develop clinical symptoms. The quotation of average intakes can, therefore, be misleading, but is useful in providing an overall picture of a population. The micronutrients most commonly reported to be lacking in the diet, i.e. consumed at levels lower than the RDA, are iron and vitamin D. Interpretation of this finding is difficult, however, since the proportion of ingested iron absorbed is inversely related to intake, and a dietary source of vitamin D may be unnecessary in people regularly exposed to sunlight. There are now some 14 trace elements known to be required by man, but for some no consensus has been reached on amounts. This is in part due to their natural abundance in most diets, and to a lack of knowledge about their bioavailability in food, and their absorption.

Interest in micronutrient deficiency has been concentrated on a few groups within the population who are regarded as being particularly vulnerable. These are immigrants, in whom a combination of dietary and cultural factors increases their risk, pregnant women, and growing children. To these groups might be added vegetarians, particularly vegans, but in most cases the concern is unjustified [4].

Non-European immigration into the United Kingdom has been predominantly from the Indian subcontinent and from the Caribbean. Immigrant families usually have a diet markedly different from the normal British diet, and first-generation immigrant women will continue to cook only according to their own customs. The nutrition of mothers, infants and children can cause special problems not exclusive to but largely confined to immigrant groups. Asian mothers are the most likely to be anaemic and deficient in vitamin D. There is a high incidence of osteomalacia in pregnant Asian women, with a high risk of fetal or neonatal rickets in their infants [5]. Rickets in children has also been encountered in almost every centre of the Asian population in the United Kingdom. The cause of this deficiency is primarily the restrictions of the traditional diet combined with a failure to synthesise adequate amounts of vitamin D due to a lack of exposure to sunlight.

Social class is an important factor influencing the quality of diet, and studies on the dietary habits of pregnant women have revealed a social class gradient for intakes of many of the micronutrients. Since the incidence of low birthweight and congenital abnormality is also class-related, much interest has recently been shown in the suggestion that deficiencies of one or more of these nutrients might contribute to those conditions. Smithells et al. [6] measured the blood concentration of a number of vitamins in the first trimester of pregnancy in over 900 women. Those from social classes I and II showed significantly higher mean levels than women of lower social class with respect to erythrocyte folate and riboflavin, leucocyte vitamin C and serum vitamin A. In this work originated the hypothesis that specific vitamin deficiencies might be involved in the causation of neural tube defects [7]. Between 60% and 70% of developmental abnormalities in man are unexplained. To date there is only circumstantial evidence that an inadequate vitamin or trace element intake may have an adverse effect in pregnancy (vitamin D excepted). In a recent study in Aberdeen, normal primigravidae were compared with primigravidae who had been assigned to a "low birthweight" category on the basis of their physical characteristics and weight gain in pregnancy. Plasma concentrations of iron, zinc and copper, together with the dietary intakes of these elements, were measured. Plasma concentrations of all three trace elements were found to be comparable in the two groups. Furthermore no correlation was noted between plasma levels and dietary intakes [8]. Meeting the needs for the macronutrients is a less controversial subject; their role in human physiology is part of nutritional history.

The composition of the average diets of 21 countries including the extremes of affluence and poverty are shown in Table 1.1. The data are abstracted from the most recent Food Balance Sheets produced by the Food and Agricultural Organisation [9]. They present a comprehensive picture of the pattern of each country's food supply for human consumption from all sources (production, imports and changes in food stocks) over a period of 3 years. They provide information on daily per head consumption of primary and processed commodities divided into foods of animal and vegetable origin, and average intakes of energy, protein and fat. For the calculations, carbohydrate was estimated "by difference". The amounts of food actually eaten are likely to be lower than the quantities shown in the Food Balance Sheets, depending on the extent of food losses and of wastage in the home – a factor impossible to predict. They will also be affected by the reliability of basic statistics of population size. Nevertheless, these data give the best estimates available for purposes of comparison.

Table 1.1. Food consumption in 21 countries ranging from the most affluent to the most impoverished. The countries are ranked in order of values for mean daily energy intakes given in the FAO Food Balance Sheets

Country	Mean daily energy intake (kcal)[a]	Source of energy (%)		
		Protein	Fat	Carbohydrate
Italy	3688	11.4	34.0	54.6
United States	3641	11.6	41.6	46.8
Hungary	3484	10.9	34.0	55.1
Great Britain	3249	11.1	39.5	49.4
Sweden	3146	11.3	42.8	45.9
Australia	3055	11.8	31.3	56.9
Japan	2852	12.4	25.4	62.2
Mean	3302	11.5	35.5	53.0
Hong Kong	2771	11.8	37.1	51.1
Chile	2759	11.0	18.6	70.4
Algeria	2586	10.2	19.7	70.1
Brazil	2578	9.2	17.8	73.0
Jamaica	2544	10.0	21.8	68.2
Philippines	2405	9.0	11.9	79.1
Sudan	2314	11.3	28.0	60.7
Mean	2565	10.4	22.1	67.5
Peru	2195	10.7	17.3	72.0
Guatemala	2138	10.9	17.3	71.8
Kenya	2011	10.8	17.4	71.8
Haiti	1905	9.6	14.3	76.1
Mali	1893	10.9	18.3	70.8
Bangladesh	1837	8.6	6.6	84.8
Ghana	1769	9.3	15.5	75.2
Mean	1964	10.1	15.2	74.7

Source: FAO Food Balance Sheets [9].
[a]Although these values appear in the Food Balance Sheets as "Mean Daily Energy Intakes", they are, in reality, estimates of food moving into consumption per head of population, with no regard to the demographic structure of the populations.

The figures suggest that when the means to purchase food and the availability of food are no longer factors that influence food choice, man intuitively selects a balance between the major nutrients (protein, fat and carbohydrate), although this may appear to have little relevance to physiological needs. The differences among the countries in the proportions of total food energy provided by these nutrients are least in the seven industrialised nations included in the table.

By far the most variable constituent of the diet is fat, which shows a six-fold difference in the extent to which it contributes energy to the diet. If mean daily energy intakes are taken into account, it will be seen that the average American consumes

12 times as much fat as the average Bangladeshi. Fat is the most obvious nutritional index of affluence. The amount of fat required by man is, however, remarkably small, and is determined primarily by his need for the polyunsaturated fatty acids, linoleic and α-linolenic acid, and for the transport of the fat-soluble vitamins from the lumen of the gut. Fatty acids other than linoleic and α-linolenic acid are continuously synthesised from carbohydrate, since the transient and long-term storage of energy in the form of carbohydrate, the major source of energy in almost all human diets, is limited.

Although the amount of energy provided by fat may fall to very low levels in the poorest of the developing countries, such as Bangladesh, essential fatty acid (EFA) deficiency arising from a dietary lack has never been described in adult man, and there is only one report of EFA deficiency occurring in young children suffering from protein-energy malnutrition [10]. It is fortuitous that, as the amount of fat habitually eaten declines, the proportion obtained from vegetable sources, which are particularly rich in polyunsaturated fatty acids, rises (Fig. 1.1). The experiments of Hansen and his colleagues on infants in which artificial milk formulas low in linoleic acid were fed suggested that linoleic acid need provide no more than 1% of the total dietary energy [11]. Later studies have indicated that the requirement might be even less, and thus would easily be met by 20 g of a vegetable oil in the diet of an adult man or

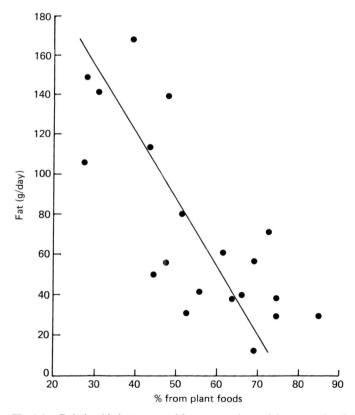

Fig. 1.1.   Relationship between total fat consumption and the proportion derived from plant foods; data from 21 different countries (see Table 1.1). $r = 0.78$, $p<0.001$.

woman [12,13]. This amount would also meet the needs for absorption of the fat-soluble vitamins. A proportion of fat well in excess of that needed to prevent EFA deficiency is, however, conducive to the achievement of an optimum energy intake.

The ingestion of foods rich in fat is responsible for the high energy density of Western diets and is believed by some to account for the high prevalence of obesity. Energy density is a term in popular use in the current debate on healthy eating, but it has not been clearly defined. It is easily understood when discussing the weaning diets of developing countries that are associated with the induction of protein energy malnutrition. For example, the traditional weaning food of the Yorubas of Western Nigeria was found on analysis to provide 0.27 kcal/g [10]. It is more difficult to apply to the complex diets of adults in industrialised populations. Should the weight of the food include the weight of beverages such as sweetened tea and coffee, fruit squashes and soft drinks which, themselves of low energy density (0.2–0.4 kcal/g) contribute substantial amounts of energy, mostly in the form of sugar, to the diet of many young adults? A more useful definition would be "energy per unit of dry weight". Using the values for the major nutrients given in the Food Balance Sheets the energy densities of the diets of the United States and of Bangladesh would be 5.20 kcal/g and 4.15 kcal/g respectively – a significant difference which would be somewhat greater were the fibre contents of the two diets to be taken into account.

The question of a specific need for carbohydrate is only of academic interest. More than half of the total dietary energy of adult men and women is normally supplied in this form, and since almost all of the dietary protein is oxidised, and thereby provides carbohydrate by the process of gluconeogenesis, even a diet that traditionally contained very little carbohydrate, such as that of the Greenland Eskimos (Table 1.2), was particularly rich in its precursor, protein [14].

It is surprising how little difference there is among the different nations of the world in the proportion of dietary energy derived from protein (Table 1.1), although the total amount consumed is directly related to calorie intake. Even in a meat-producing country such as Argentina, which has a high per head energy intake (3380 kcal/day) protein represents on average 13.3% of the total food energy [9]. The notion that these figures indicate an innate preference for a balance of protein and energy around 10%, given that many individual foods readily available in the markets of the richer nations have a much higher ratio, is an appealing one. Average values for protein concentration in the diet can, however, be misleading. Groups within any population must inevitably eat more than average and others less. There is a widely held view amongst nutritionists that protein in some way regulates its own consumption, although evidence for this belief from adequately controlled human studies is regrettably sparse [15,16,17].

In a metabolic study designed to establish whether nitrogen equilibrium could be maintained in overweight volunteers fed a 1000-kcal diet (Naismith and Holdsworth, unpublished data) it was noted that when protein provided 50% of the total energy the subjects had difficulty in consuming their meals, although these were varied, extremely palatable and prepared from normal food items (veal, fillet steak, non-oily fish and chicken). Furthermore they did not experience hunger at any time during the 6-week period of study. When the concentration of protein was reduced to 14%, appetite and hunger promptly returned. Attempts have been made in experiments on rats to explain the apparent regulatory effect of protein on food consumption. The hypothesis tested was that the ingestion of protein affects the plasma "tryptophan ratio" (the ratio of tryptophan to the aromatic and branched chain amino acids that share a common carrier that transports the amino acids into the tissues, including the brain) and consequently the uptake of tryptophan by the brain and the synthesis of the neurotransmitter serotonin. Although the administration of tryptophan alone or the feeding of unusual mixtures of amino acids designed to alter the plasma tryptophan ratio were found to alter serotonin synthesis in acute experiments, no connection between chronic dietary protein intake and serotonin synthesis was found [18].

Table 1.2. Composition of the traditional diet of Greenland Eskimos and of modern Greenlanders (expressed as a percentage of total food energy)

	Protein	Fat	Carbohydrate
Traditional 2559 kcal/day	44.1	47.5	8.4
Modern 3544 kcal/day	29.8	18.4	51.8

Source: Sinclair [14].

High levels of protein consumption are usually associated with high total energy intakes. Man can, however, adapt to much greater intakes of protein when his natural environment provides predominantly animal foods. The most striking example is the Eskimo. Sinclair has had a life-long fascination with the eating habits of Eskimos [14]. Eskimos live mainly near the coast, and formerly obtained most of their food from the sea. The supply was seasonal. The main food throughout the hungry winter was seal, procured with unbelievable hardship and ingenuity. Later in the year walrus, narwhal, occasionally polar bear, caribou, small rodents and fish were eaten. In summer the Eskimo enjoyed a more abundant omnivorous diet, when a variety of berries, roots and leaves became available. The composition of the traditional diet is shown in Table 1.2. It contained the highest proportions of protein and fat of any human diet described. Much of the limited intake of carbohydrate was derived from animal tissue glycogen reserves.

The original Eskimo was adapted very efficiently to life as a carnivore, and there is no evidence that consumption of so much protein was detrimental to his health or was the cause of his relatively low energy intake. Contact with Western man has, however, radically altered the balance of his diet. The modern Greenlander still consumes an unusually large amount of protein, derived mainly from fish, but the carbohydrate intake, from the purchase of flour and sugar, falls within the range of intakes of most prosperous countries, and fat intake is relatively low. In a return to his study of the Eskimo, Sinclair [19] ate for 100 days a typical Eskimo diet composed entirely of marine animal foods: seal, fish, crustaceans and molluscs. Although his interest was then in blood lipids and in haemostasis he noted that the lack of carbohydrate foods, as discussed earlier, presented no problem. Ketonuria was not detectable even after prolonged physical exercise.

It is axiomatic that the need for protein is greatest at times of rapid growth when, in addition to maintaining existing tissues, new tissue is being manufactured and, in the case of the young baby, tissue maturation is taking place. The ideal diet for the human infant is generally acknowledged to be breast milk, a product that combines the maximum efficiency of utilisation with the promotion of optimum growth. The composition of breast milk, based on the analyses of pooled samples from five regions of the United Kingdom [20] is shown in Table 1.3. No more then 6.1% of the total energy is provided in the form of protein, yet this low concentration permits the doubling of birthweight in under 5 months. The proportional requirements of adult man for protein of similar quality must obviously be less, and, even allowing for the lower biological value of protein in a mixed diet, would remain well below 10%. But pragmatic rather than scientific arguments have prevailed, and those charged with making dietary recommendations [21] have endorsed customary dietary practices. A low-protein diet would be unpalatable and monotonous to the privileged Westerner; to the Bangladeshi it is simply a fact of life.

Table 1.3. Composition (per 100 ml) of human milk and of a typical unmodified cow's milk formula

	Protein		Fat		Carbohydrate	
	g	% energy	g	% energy	g	% energy
Human milk	1.07	6.1	4.2	54.1	7.4	39.7
Formula	3.00	18.4	3.9	53.9	4.8	27.6

Source: DHSS [20].

A Balanced Diet for Growth

As in all mammals, growth in man begins in the uterus, where an appropriate balance of nutrients is selected from the maternal circulation for active transport to the fetus. The exception is the supply of glucose, the unique fuel of the growing fetus which, since glucose crosses the placenta by a process of facilitated diffusion, is susceptible to the vagaries of the maternal blood concentration.

The fasting glucose concentration, with which the body functions throughout most of the day, is slightly reduced from early pregnancy and is homeostatically regulated. There are, however, circumstances in which it can be altered. A small proportion of healthy women show diabetic responses in the course of pregnancy which revert to normal after delivery. The transient abnormally high concentrations of glucose in the blood after meals increase the transfer of glucose to the fetus and so induce fat synthesis. The infants are usually overweight. Normal birthweight data show that about 3% of mothers give birth to infants weighing more than 4.5 kg [22]. More common (around 6%) is the underweight infant, weighing less than 2.5 kg, the product of an inadequate energy supply.

Energy is the prime determinant of fetal growth. Intervention studies on chronically undernourished women have shown no benefit to the fetus from protein supplementation. Energy supplements, on the other hand, have produced significant improvements in growth; the greater the dietary deficit, the greater was the increase in birthweight, but the effect was limited. Lechtig and Klein [23] describe an "energy threshold" of around 1600–1700 kcal/day, beyond which supplementation has no appreciable effect. This amount of food would generally be regarded as barely adequate for a non-gravid woman within the same community. Studies on the dietary behaviour of healthy pregnant women in well-nourished populations have clarified this rather confusing observation. On average, women do not appreciably alter their customary food intake during pregnancy [24]. The additional costs of pregnancy are met by making adjustments in the absorption, excretion and metabolism of the nutrients. Poor growth of the fetus can therefore arise from a lack of energy (glucose) in the maternal diet. Alternatively, competition from the muscles for glucose during periods of hard physical work in women who, through poverty, are unable to raise their level of food consumption, can also lead to low birthweight [25].

There is no evidence that the balance of nutrients in the optimal diet of a young woman need be altered during pregnancy, or that the choice of food is spontaneously changed other than in response to cravings for or an aversion to certain foods. These peculiarities of appetite have no nutritional basis, and are thought to arise from alterations in the threshold for all forms of taste: salt, sweet, sour and bitter.

Concern about the diet of pregnant women in developed countries, particularly those who had been judged to have a poor diet (i.e. who failed to meet the recommended allowances for reproduction) has led, in some instances, to the use of high-protein supplements, protein being perceived to have particular importance for fetal growth [26–30]. While well intentioned, these feeding trials did not have the effects intended. High-protein supplements were claimed to be associated with a depression rather than an increase in birthweight and in length and [30] with increased very early pre-term delivery and neonatal death, whereas balanced or low-protein supplements produced modest increases in birthweight averaging about 50 g [31]. Grieve et al. [32] have described the remarkable effects of a high-protein diet on birthweight in Motherwell, Scotland. In the practice of one consultant obstetrician a diet very high in animal protein and low in carbohydrate was routinely prescribed for many years. Comparison of the Motherwell records with those for a population similar in stature and in socio-economic background in Aberdeen revealed a deficit in birthweight of more than 400 g. This deficit is comparable to that observed in times of famine.

Although higher than average intakes of protein may be tolerated in healthy men and women, high levels of consumption seem to disturb the optimum balance of nutrients required during pregnancy, with detrimental effects on fetal growth and on the viability of the neonate. The mechanism of this effect is not understood, but low birthweight probably results from the reduction of total energy intake rather than from a specific effect of protein.

An excessive intake of protein can also influence growth postnatally. The ideal diet for the newborn infant is generally acknowledged to be breast milk. In the early 1970s a number of reports appeared in the medical literature describing abnormally rapid growth in infants, accompanied by a high incidence of overweight [33,34,35]. This was associated with the decline in breast feeding at that time (see Fig. 1.4). The abnormal weight gain was attributed to excessive energy intakes from bottle feeds and to the practice of introducing cereal weaning foods at too early an age. Inaccuracies in the preparation of feeds and encouragement of infants to consume more milk than they would voluntarily have taken from the breast were thought to be responsible.

It seemed to us [36] more likely, however, that the cause of accelerated growth in these infants was their high intake of protein rather than of energy: Fomon [37] had demonstrated convincingly that infants can regulate their energy intakes, the volume of artificial milk consumed by his infant subjects varying inversely with the energy density of the feed so that total energy intake was not changed. Furthermore the cereal foods commonly used to initiate weaning contained considerably more protein than does breast milk. The most popular artificial feeds in the early 1970s were simply dried cow's milk to which vitamins had been added. Although, when properly constituted, the milks provided the same concentration of energy as does breast milk (around 70 kcal/100 ml), they contained almost three times as much protein (Table 1.3).

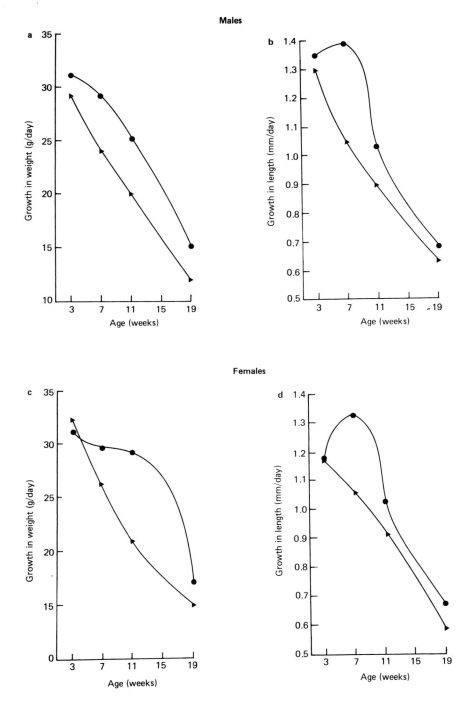

Fig. 1.2. Rates of growth in weight and in length of 10 male (**a** and **b**) and 10 female (**c** and **d**) infants. *Triangles*, breast-fed infants; *circles*, infants fed on high-protein formula.

Table 1.4.   Rates of growth in weight (g/day) and in length (mm/day) of breast-fed and formula-fed infants

	Male (n = 10)		Female (n = 10)	
	g/day	mm/day	g/day	mm/day
Breast-fed	27.1	1.09	24.8	1.06
Low-protein formula	26.9	1.17	25.0	1.12
High-protein formula	33.3	1.26	29.8	1.18

Source: Naismith and Ritchie [36].

We tested the hypothesis by comparing the rate of growth, in weight and in length, of 20 breast-fed infants with the rate in two groups of 20 infants who were formula-fed. One formula-fed group received a typical high-protein milk, the other a "humanised" formula with a protein concentration similar to that of breast milk. Milk intakes were recorded. The rates of gain in both weight and height were virtually identical in the breast-fed infants and those fed the low-protein formula. Infants on the high-protein formula, however, showed a striking acceleration in their rate of growth ending the 3-month study 22% heavier and 13% longer than the breast-fed infants. Average daily energy intakes did not differ significantly between the formula-fed groups. It was concluded that the high concentration of protein in the unmodified cow's milk formula was the sole cause of the acceleration in growth (Table 1.4). Growth velocity curves (Fig. 1.2) showed that in breast-fed infants the rate of growth in weight and in length declines steadily from birth. This also occurred in the formula-fed infants on the high-protein formula, but at all stages the rate of growth in this group was always greater. In the female infants the distortion of the normal pattern of growth was particularly evident.

Although our study lasted for 4 months only, it is likely that with the continued use of high-protein milks and fortified cereals accelerated growth would continue for much longer. One weaning food in common use at the time contained 46% protein. Whether increased growth velocity in infancy and early childhood will have adverse consequences in later life is open to question. All that can be said, at present, is that it is unnatural, if by "natural" we mean the mode of growth displayed by the suckling-infant. It is now recognised that poor growth in children in developing countries is due to a deficiency of energy, i.e. total food, rather than to deficiency of a specific nutrient, such as protein. The demonstration that growth could be normalised in children suffering from moderate protein-energy malnutrition by supplementing their simple cereal-based diet with more of the same laid the ghost of the "protein gap" that dominated nutritional thinking in the 1960s.

In industrialised countries secular changes in the heights and weights of children are believed to reflect general improvements in medical care, in social well-being, and particularly in nutrition, commensurate with the progressive rise in prosperity. In all Western countries, however, underprivileged groups still persist within the population whose standards of health and nutrition are regarded as unsatisfactory. Poor children are in general shorter than average, though not necessarily lighter, and tend to consume a monotonous diet, borderline in its adequacy [38].

Concern about the growth and development of poor inner-city children prompted us to investigate the relationship between growth, diet and social background [39]. Between 1973 and 1976, 1000 households randomly selected from poor areas in London were surveyed. Census indicators of urban deprivation such as overcrowding, lack of basic amenities, unemployment, and a high proportion of the population under the age of 14 years were used in the selection. Two hundred and thirty-one "at risk" children from 112 families were identified, the criteria for classification being households headed by single parents, four or more dependent children below the age of 12, overcrowding, and total dependence on Supplementary Benefit (an extra allowance for poor families provided by the British Social Security system). For all children between the ages of 1 and 12 in each family, records were made of food intake over a 3-day period, and heights and weights, triceps and subscapular skinfold thicknesses, and mid-upper arm circumferences were measured.

Twenty-one per cent of the children fell below the 10th percentile for height, and a larger proportion than expected were at the "light" end of the weight distribution. Dietary data for the shorter children, at or below the 10th percentile for height or with siblings at or below the 10th percentile, showed levels of nutrient intakes below the average for the group as a whole. The intake of energy was only 72% of the RDA [40], but intakes of protein, calcium, vitamins A and C, and the B vitamins all met or exceeded recommended values. The only nutrient that might give cause for concern was iron (80% of the RDA). The lack of dietary energy was again seen to be the single most probable cause of growth failure, a conclusion confirmed by the views of the parents. Of those who believed their children's diets to be unsatisfactory, most complained of lack of quantity as a consequence of inadequate income.

Current disquiet about the nutrition of British children is focussed on an alleged imbalance between wholesome natural foods and processed foods in their largely self-selected meals. The term "junk food", a fabrication of the mass media, is a pejorative one frequently used to characterise the diet of the average young adolescent. There is clearly no such commodity as a junk food. Anything eaten that provides energy is a food. Sugar, which provides energy alone, may be the sole constituent of some forms of confectionery. It is not difficult, however, to think of circumstances in which such confectionery would be both useful and convenient. A food that contains nutrients in appreciable amounts in addition to energy might be more beneficial if the diet as a whole were believed to be borderline or deficient in specific nutrients. As mentioned earlier, the value of any item in the diet depends on how often it is eaten, and in what quantity. It would be surprising if the average diet of young people living in the United Kingdom were indeed lacking in nutrients when our study [39] revealed no significant deficiencies in the country's most deprived community.

On the recommendation of the Committee on Medical Aspects of Food Policy (COMA) a survey was commissioned by the Department of Health and Social Security (DHSS), the British Government Ministry of Health, as part of its responsibility for monitoring the effects of national food policy. A preliminary report has been published [41]. A nationally representative sample of children drawn from maintained schools in England, Wales and Scotland recorded all food and drink consumed over 7 days. Heights and weights were measured, and a socio-economic questionnaire was administered. Full information was provided on 3285 children. The children fell into two groups: 10–11-year-olds and 14–15-year-olds. Although it is well known that the age of onset of puberty in both boys and girls is very variable, it was hoped that the younger sample would contain predominantly girls who had not reached menarche, and the older sample boys who had entered their adolescent growth spurt.

The results of the dietary analyses were reported as average consumptions of 38 different groups of food and as average intakes of energy and nutrients. Comparisons were made with the RDAs defined by the DHSS [21]. The RDAs for nutrients are designed to ensure that in a group of healthy people the requirements of almost all will be met. They are based on mean requirements to which a generous margin of safety is added. Consequently most individuals will have requirements less than the RDAs, some considerably less. The recommendations for energy, however, are, for obvious reasons, based on mean intakes of different groups within a healthy population.

In the diets of the children surveyed protein, on average, accounted for 12% of the energy intake in all groups, thus exceeding the RDA (Table 1.5). Intakes of calcium, vitamins A and C, and the B vitamins (thiamin, riboflavin and niacin) all met or surpassed the RDAs. Only in the case of iron were intakes below recommended values in all children except the older boys. Normally about 10% of dietary iron is absorbed, but when intakes fall, the efficiency of absorption is increased. The report concluded that most of the children were likely to be absorbing sufficient iron, but that some of the older girls, particularly those on slimming diets, were likely to be at risk.

Contrary to popular opinion, the average diets were varied and wholesome, as confirmed by the nutrient analyses. Dairy products featured prominently, accounting for the high intakes of calcium, and fruit and vegetables made an important contribution to all diets, although potatoes in various forms (including chips and crisps) alone would satisfy the needs for vitamin C. Crisps and corn snacks provided on average 4% only of the total energy, and confectionery 6%.

Table 1.5. Mean daily intakes of energy and nutrients of British schoolchildren (Recommended Daily Allowances shown in parentheses)

	Age 10–11		Age 14–15	
	Boys	Girls	Boys	Girls
Energy (kcal)	2070 (2270)	1840 (2030)	2490 (2750)	1880 (2150)
Protein (g)	61.0 (57)	53.2 (51)	74.6 (66)	56.2 (53)
Calcium (mg)	833 (700)	702 (700)	925 (650	692 (650)
Iron (mg)	10.0 (12)	8.6 (12)	12.2 (12)	9.3 (12)
Vitamin C (mg)	49.3 (25)	49.0 (25)	49.3 (28)	48.0 (28)
Vitamin A (µg)	854 (575)	691 (575)	969 (750)	801 (750)
Thiamin (mg)	1.21 (0.9)	1.03 (0.8)	1.47 (1.1)	1.04 (0.9)
Riboflavin (mg)	1.70 (1.2)	1.40 (1.2)	1.89 (1.5)	1.32 (1.5)
Niacin (mg)	26.5 (14)	23.1 (14)	32.6 (18)	24.0 (18)

Source: Wenlock et al. [41].

Children receiving sufficient energy to meet their requirements for growth would be expected to have reached the standards for height and weight in British children devised by Tanner and his colleagues in 1965 [42]. Average energy intakes in both groups of children were found to be about 10% below the RDA. There was, however, no evidence of undernutrition. The findings for the 10–11-year-olds are shown in Fig. 1.3. On average boys weighed nearly 5 kg and girls 4 kg more than their counterparts in 1965. These increments in weight have been claimed by some to reflect a decline in physical activity in British children during the past two decades. Such an explanation might reconcile the conflicting evidence of excessive weight gain and a deficit in energy intake, but would not explain the increase in height recorded in these children. Average height in both sexes was 3.5 cm greater than in 1965. The picture was similar in the 14–15-year-olds, although at this age the differences from standard values, particularly in the girls, were much reduced.

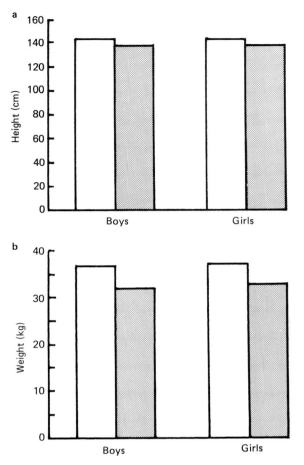

Fig. 1.3. Average heights (**a**) and weights (**b**) of 10–11-year-old children measured in 1985 (*open columns*) compared with 1965 standards (*stippled columns*).

An acceleration in the rate of growth is, *inter alia*, a consequence of an improvement in nutritional status of the population. In Europe and North America these trends continued at a steady pace until the 1960s, when a slowing down was noted [43]. It is assumed that children are now able to achieve their optimal growth potential.

Associated with accelerated growth the timing of puberty is advanced. It has long been known that poor nutrition delays sexual development in boys and girls. Over the last 100 years there has been a progressive trend to earlier menarche in girls of around 3–4 months per decade in Europe [44]. Thus the timing of puberty is controlled by some factor other than chronological age. During childhood the rate of gain in weight averages 2.5 kg per year in well-nourished populations. At the onset of puberty, around the age of 10 for girls and 12 for boys, the velocity of growth in weight is increased. Growth velocity in height follows a similar pattern, coincident but to a lesser degree. Although the adolescent growth spurt contributes almost 50% to young adult body weight, the linear spurt contributes only 15% to final adult height [45]. Thus an earlier onset of puberty would entail a more striking increase in body weight than in height, as observed in the 10–11-year-olds in the DHSS survey [41].

The nature of the increments in weight at the time of maximum growth velocity is different in boys compared with girls. The body composition of children is similar, fat representing about 12% of total body mass, but accretion of fat in girls begins 3–4 years before menarche, so that, at the time of peak velocity in growth the proportion of fat has risen to 19%, and at menarche, one year later, to 24% [46]. The ratio of lean body weight to fat therefore changes during sexual development from 5 : 1 at the initiation of the growth spurt to 3 : 1 at menarche. In growing adolescent boys no such change occurs. Frisch [46] has observed that menarche and the maintenance of regular ovulatory cycles in women appear to depend on reaching and maintaining a minimum weight for height. Since fat is the most variable component of the body, responding rapidly to changes in energy balance, Frisch has postulated that a critical ratio of body fat to lean tissue is an important determinant for reproductive ability in young women. This idea makes sound physiological sense. Adipose tissue may be a significant extra-gonadal source of oestrogens [47]. Furthermore the body fat store of a healthy young woman represents an energy reserve of some 120 000 kcal, an amount sufficient to assure the additional energy cost of pregnancy, estimated at about 80 000 kcal [48], and provide a generous subsidy towards the high energy cost of lactation.

The major aim of the reports of both the National Advisory Committee on Nutrition Education, NACNE [1] and the Committee on the Medical Aspects of Food Policy, COMA [49] on diet and health is a reduction in the proportion of total food energy derived from fat, the target suggested for healthier eating being 35% or less. Only about one quarter of the boys and one fifth of the girls in both age groups of the DHSS sample could therefore be classified as healthy eaters. A substantial proportion of the boys, and even more of the girls, obtained between 40% and 50% of their total calories from fat (Table 1.6). This observation raises some important questions: is there an innate preference or need for high-energy foods during periods of rapid growth and vigorous lifestyle? The suckling infant receives around 50% of its energy intake from fat (Table 1.3). Does the selection of high-fat foods by girls in particular reflect an inherent drive to attain a body composition conducive to fertility? Would the healthier diet proposed for consumption by our overweight, physically inactive adult population, with the prime purpose of reducing the incidence of death from coronary heart disease, constitute a balanced diet for young teenagers? Although these ideas are highly speculative, as is the notion that the dietary habits of young

Table 1.6.   Daily intake of fat of British schoolchildren as a proportion of total dietary energy

Age	Fat (% energy)	Boys (%)	Girls (%)
10–11	35.1–40.0	56	52
	40.1–45.0	18	27
	45.1–50.0	2	1
14–15	35.1–40.0	49	47
	40.1–45.0	25	34
	45.1–50.0	3	3

Source: Wenlock et al. [41].

teenagers set an immutable pattern for adult life, they none the less cast doubt on the general prescription of the "healthier diet" for all groups of the population.

Further speculation is needed on the unexpected increase in average heights and weights of children that is apparent in the 1983 sample [41] when compared with the 1965 standards [42], particularly since government intervention in the diets of children was lessened during their lifetime, and no notable improvement in nutritional standards over the last 20 years has been recognised. A clue might be found in their earlier nutritional experience. The children participating in the DHSS survey were born in the late sixties and early seventies. At that time the practice of breast feeding had declined to its nadir. Figure 1.4 depicts the change that has occurred in the incidence of breast feeding over the 40 years in a major maternity hospital in Edinburgh [50]. This picture is not atypical [51]. The great majority of infants in the late sixties and early seventies were fed high-protein unmodified cow's milk formulas such as National Dried Milk and similar proprietary brands, which have been found to accelerate growth in infancy, and received early supplementary feeding with protein-enriched weaning foods. The critical question is whether the increment in growth arising in infancy would be maintained in later childhood. There is some evidence to support such a proposition.

Figure 1.5 is reproduced from the Fourth Boyd Orr Memorial Lecture given by A. M. Thomson [52]. It illustrates the changes in average heights of successive cohorts of London schoolboys measured between 1905 and 1959. It is noteworthy that almost 60% of the gain in height at the age of 13, some 13 cm over 50 years, is accounted for by the difference in height at the age of 5. Overnutrition in infancy could therefore influence both height and weight in adolescence, probably by advancing the onset of sexual development. Whether average adult stature will ultimately be affected remains to be discovered. It may be that maximum linear growth within the limits imposed by genetics has already been reached in most industrialised countries, although social class differences remain, and are unlikely to be genetic in origin. Thomson [52] has suggested that achieving maximum linear growth is desirable for optimum physiological efficiency, and cites as evidence in support of his

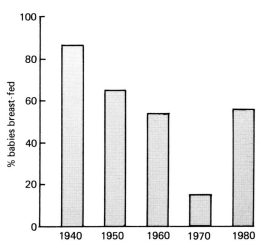

Fig. 1.4. Changes in the prevalence of breast feeding over a 40-year period in a major hospital (Simpson Memorial Maternity Pavilion, Edinburgh).

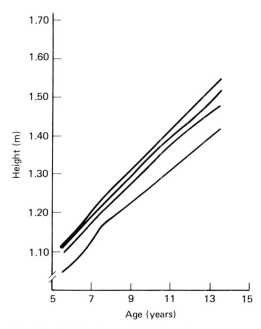

Fig. 1.5. Secular changes in heights of London schoolboys from 1905–12 to 1959 [52].

hypothesis that obstetric disability is much less in tall women, and that the risk of coronary heart disease is less in tall men than in short men. Although there is no evidence that accelerating growth is either beneficial to health or poses a risk to health, it has, however, been suggested that earlier maturation might lead to earlier development of degenerative diseases or even to a shorter lifespan [1].

Should the DHSS in 10 years' time repeat its survey of British schoolchildren, this time on a generation nurtured at the breast or on "humanised" infant feeds, young adolescents may be found to be shorter and lighter than their 1983 counterparts, and health educators will again decry their dietary habits.

A Balanced Diet for Optimum Health

The total amount of energy that would be provided from meeting the minimum needs for fat and protein would be no more than 400 kcal per day. Does it matter from what food sources the additional 2000 kcal consumed by an adult man or woman is derived? This question has been addressed by various official and unofficial bodies concerned with evaluating the long-term effects of diet composition on health and with offering guidance to the public and to the food manufacturers. Inspection of Table 1.1 shows that different countries go about providing these calories in different ways, the major differences in gross composition of their average diets being related to their degree of economic prosperity. With decreasing affluence total energy intake may fall and energy from fat is replaced with energy from carbohydrate. Furthermore there are important changes in the quality of the diet. The proportion of fat of animal origin falls with increasing poverty, and the proportion of complex carbohydrates (starch and dietary fibre) rises at the expense of simple sugars, mostly sucrose.

Ironically the diet of poverty sets the standards for healthy eating. A reduction in total fat intake with a higher ratio of polyunsaturated to saturated fatty acids is advocated with the object of lowering the incidence of cardiovascular disease in general, and coronary heart disease in particular [1,49]. The resulting decrease in the energy density of the diet, it is believed, would facilitate weight loss in the obese. A restriction in sugar consumption is encouraged with a view to reducing the incidence of dental caries and obesity, and the substitution of fibre-rich carbohydrate (from bread, cereals, fruit and vegetables) for part of the fat is recommended on the basis of the alleged beneficial properties of fibre. These are said to be in reducing the risk of heart disease, lowering the plasma cholesterol concentration, modulating glucose absorption and preventing large bowel disease. With the aim of reducing hypertensive disease, a major risk factor in the development of both coronary heart disease and cerebrovascular disease, a reduction in the use of salt has also been suggested.

In matters of nutritional education, Government usually demands a very high standard of proof on which to base its policies but, for pragmatic reasons, must often settle for less, making recommendations in accordance with the best current scientific opinion. Others are less demanding. The recommendations are intended for the population as a whole, with exclusion of the under-fives. This is no doubt in the public interest. Although it is well known that there is a wide variability in response to dietary modification within the population, the alternative – to identify and target those most likely to benefit from an alteration in their dietary habits such as the obese, the hypertensive and those with elevated blood cholesterol – would be prohibitively expensive. It is important, however, to recognise that the "healthful diet" may not always provide the optimum balance of nutrients for all sections of the population.

References

1. NACNE (1983) A discussion paper on proposals for nutritional guidelines for health education in Britain. Health Education Council, London
2. WHO (1968) Nutritional anaemias. Technical report series 405. WHO, Rome
3. Davies CTM, Chukweumeka AC,van Haaren JPM (1973) Iron deficiency anaemia: its effect on maximum aerobic power and responses to exercise in African males aged 17–40 years. Clin Sci 44:555–562
4. Sanders TAB, Key TJA (1987) Blood pressure, plasma renin activity and aldosterone concentrations in vegans and omnivore controls, Hum Nutr Appl Nutr 41A:204–211
5. Dunnigan MG, Smith CM (1965) The aetiology of late rickets in Pakistani children in Glasgow – report of a diet survey. Scott Med J 10:1–9
6. Smithells RW, Sheppard S, Schorah CJ (1976) Vitamin deficiencies and neural tube defects. Arch Dis Child 51:944–950
7. Dobbing J (1983) prevention of spina bifida and other neural tube defects. Academic Press, London
8. Tuttle S (1982) Trace element requirements during pregnancy. In: Campbell DM, Gillmer MDG (eds) Nutrition in pregnancy. Royal College of Obstetricians and Gynaecologists, London, pp 47–54
9. FAO (1984) Food balance sheets (1979–1981 average). FAO, Rome
10. Naismith DJ (1973) Kwashiorkor in Western Nigeria: a dietary study with particular reference to energy and linoleic acid. Br J Nutr 30:567–576
11. Hansen AE, Haggard ME, Boelsche AN, Adam DJD, Wiese HF (1958) Essential fatty acids in infant nutrition. III. Clinical manifestations of linoleic acid deficiency. J Nutr 66:565–576

12. Naismith DJ, Deeprose SP, Supramaniam G, Williams MJH (1978) A reappraisal of the linoleic acid requirement of the young infant, with particular regard to the use of modified cow's milk formulae. Arch Dis Child 53:845–849
13. Sanders TAB, Naismith DJ (1979) A comparison of the influence of breast feeding and bottle feeding on the fatty acid composition of the erythrocytes. Br J Nutr 41:619–623
14. Sinclair HM (1953) The diet of Canadian Indians and Eskimos. Proc Nutr Soc 12:69–82
15. Booth DA, Chase A, Campbell AT (1970) Relative effectiveness of protein in the late stages of appetite suppression in man. Physiol Behav 5:1299–1302
16. Wade J, Milner J, Krandl M (1981) Evidence for a physiological regulation of food selection and nutrient intake in twins. Am J Clin Nutr 34:143–147
17. Sunkin S, Garrow JS (1982) The satiety value of protein. Hum Nutr 36A:197–201
18. Fernstrom JD (1986) Effects of protein and carbohydrate ingestion on brain tryptophon levels and serotonin synthesis: putative relationship to appetite for specific nutrients. In: Kare MR, Brand JG (eds) Interaction of the chemical senses with nutrition. Academic press, New York pp 395–414
19. Sinclair HM (1980) Advantages and disadvantages of an Eskimo diet. In: Fumagalli R, Kritchevsky D, Paoletti R (eds) Drugs affecting lipid metabolism. Elsevier, Amsterdam
20. DHSS (1977) The composition of mature human milk. Report on health and social subjects 12. HMSO, London
21. DHSS (1979) Recommended daily amounts of food energy and nutrients for groups of people in the United Kingdom. Report on health and social subjects 15. HMSO, London
22. Thomson AM, Billewicz WZ, Hytten FE (1968) The assessment of fetal growth. J Obstet Gynaecol Br Commonwealth 75:903–916
23. Lechtig A, Klein RE (1980) Pre-natal nutrition and birthweight: is there a causal association? In: Dobbing J (ed) Maternal nutrition in pregnancy: eating for two. Academic Press, London, p 131
24. Naismith DJ (1983) Maternal nutrition and fetal health. In: Chiswick ML (ed) Recent advances in perinatal medicine 1. Churchill Livingstone, Edinburgh, pp 21–39
25. Tafari N, Naeye RL, Gobezie A (1980) Effects of maternal undernutrition and heavy physical work during pregnancy on birthweight. Br J Obstet Gynaecol 87:222–226
26. Ebbs JH, Tisdall FF, Scott WA (1941) The influence of prenatal diet on the mother and child. J Nutr 22:515–526
27. Osofsky HJ (1975) Relationships between prenatal medical and nutritional measures, pregnancy outcome, and early infant development in an urban poverty setting. I. The rate of nutritional intake. Am J Obstet Gynecol 123:682–690
28. Adams SO, Barr CD, Huenemann RL (1978) Effect of nutritional supplementation in pregnancy. I. Outcome of pregnancy. J Am Diet Assoc 72:144–147
29. Campbell-Brown M, MacGillivray I, Campbell D (1978) Energy and protein intake related to baby birthweight. Developmental Pathology Society, Aberdeen
30. Rush D, Stein Z, Susser M (1980) A randomized controlled trial of prenatal nutritional supplementation in New York City. Pediatrics 65:683–697
31. Rush D (1983) Effects of protein and calorie supplementation during pregnancy on the fetus and developing child. In: Campbell DM, Gillmer MDG (eds) Nutrition in pregnancy. Royal College of Obstetricians and Gynaecologists, London, pp 65–83
32. Grieve JFK, Campbell-Brown M, Johnstone FD (1979) Dieting in pregnancy: a study of the effect of a high protein low carbohydrate diet on birthweight and on an obstetric population. In: Sutherland MW, Stowers JM (eds) Carbohydrate metabolism in pregnancy and the newborn. Springer-Verlag, Berlin, pp 518–533
33. Taitz LS (1971) Infantile overnutrition among artificially fed infants in the Sheffield region. Br Med J i:315–316
34. Shukla A, Forsyth HA, Anderson CM, Morwah SM (1972) Infantile overnutrition in the first year of life: a field study in Dudley, Worcestershire. Br Med J iv:507–515
35. Oates RK (1973) Infant feeding practices. Br Med J ii:762–764
36. Naismith DJ, Ritchie CD (1975) A comparison of growth in wholly breast-fed infants and in artificially fed infants. Proc Nutr Soc 34:118A
37. Fomon SF (1974) Infant nutrition, 2nd ed. Saunders, Philadelphia, p 29
38. Jacoby A, Altman DG, Cook J, Holland WW, Elliott A (1975) Influence of some social and environmental factors on the nutrient intake and nutritional status of schoolchildren. Br J Prev Soc Med 29:116–120
39. Nelson M, Naismith DJ (1979) Nutritional status of poor children in London. J Hum Nutr 33:33–45
40. DHSS (1969) Recommended intakes of nutrients for the United Kingdom. Reports on health and medical subjects 120. HMSO, London

41. Wenlock RW, Disselduff MM, Skinner RB, Knight I (1986) The diets of British schoolchildren. DHSS, London
42. Tanner JM, Whitehouse RH, Takaishi M (1966) Standard from birth to maturity for height, weight, height velocity and weight velocity: British children 1965. Arch Dis Child 41:454, 613
43. Billewicz WZ, Fellowes M, Thomson AM (1981) Pubertal changes in boys and girls in Newcastle-upon-Tyne, Ann Hum Biol 8:211–219
44. Tanner JM (1962) Growth and adolescence, 2nd edn. Blackwell, Oxford
45. McLaren DS, Burman D (1976) Textbook of paediatric nutrition. Churchill Livingstone, Edinburgh
46. Frisch R (1984) Body fat, puberty and fertility. Biol Rev 59:161–188
47. Nimrod A, Ryan KJ (1975) Aromatization of androgens by human abdominal and breast fat tissue. J Clin Endocrinol Metab 40:367–372
48. Hytten FE (1980) Nutrition. In: Hytten FE, Chamberlain G (eds) Clinical physiology in obstetrics. Blackwell, Oxford, pp 165–192
49. DHSS (1984) Diet and cardiovascular disease. Reports on health and social subjects. HMSO, London
50. Belton NR (1985) Infant nutrition 1974–1984: a decade of change. In: Infant physiology and nutrition – the first year. Part I. Gardiner-Caldwell Communications, Macclesfield, pp 9–16
51. DHSS (1974) Present day practice in infant feeding. Report on health and social subjects 9. HMSO, London
52. Thomson AM (1978) Problems and politics in nutritional surveillance. Proc Nutr Soc 37:317–332

Commentary

Sanders: Naismith has side-stepped the issue of what practical advice nutritionists should give about diet, and gives the impression that it is very difficult to select an unbalanced diet. The issue at stake is not whether the majority eat well but why certain minorities eat badly. Average values hide minorities. For example, although the gross national product is high in the UK there is still poverty. Do poor-quality foods make up the diets of these minorities, and if they do, why is this so? Why is it that the unemployed and manual working classes drink and smoke more and consume a less healthy diet than higher social classes? Is it because these are the few remaining pleasures left to them?

Thomas: Naismith has rightly pointed out that although the term "balanced diet" is widely used, it is not easy to define. If we consider Bingham's suggestion, some of these difficulties become apparent. His definition of a balanced diet is one "which prevents deficiency diseases and which sustains a healthy, vigorous life. That is, a diet which contains all the essential nutrients in the optimum proportion for the individual" [1]. While this definition captures the spirit of the concept, it can be argued that, like the WHO definition of health, it does not provide easily manageable yardsticks against which a particular diet can be measured.

Levels of particular nutrients sufficient to prevent frank deficiency diseases can, and have been, measured under experimental conditions, but appropriate intakes for optimum health and avoidance of functional impairment at a more subtle level are much harder to determine and are subject to considerable scientific argument, as the case of vitamin C illustrates. In addition the interaction of nutrients provides a further complicating factor in setting desirable levels of intake for any single nutrient. Clearly, in this definition individual factors such as age, sex and activity have also to be considered in the identification of optimum proportions, and yet in some cases, such as that of the growing child as discussed by Naismith, the most desirable outcome is not at all certain, since the benefits and hazards of varying rates of growth and final size are not yet clear.

Trying to set measurable targets to fit this definition has something of the uncertainty of ten-pin bowling with invisible pins. Perhaps this is one reason why the contributors to this book have addressed the relationship between diet and disease rather than that between diet and health.

Reference

1. Bingham S (1977) Dictionary of nutrition. Barrie and Jenkins, London

Sanders: There is considerable controversy as to whether early sexual maturation is desirable. Early age of menarche is associated with increased risk of breast cancer, and in experimental animals rapid growth is associated with a shorter lifespan.

Dobbing: I agree with Thomas and Sanders that we cannot define optimum growth. The idea that it is synonymous with maximum *proper* growth is probably a better one than any which advocates growth restriction. In the absence of a definition of "proper", which would include a target of normal body composition for each age such as to exclude, for example, obesity, I suspect that a maximum rate of growth in body length, or height, would be a sensible index and a good target.

Would Sanders advocate later menarche because he says early menarche is associated with breast cancer? How? And can he envisage advising the avoidance of obesity so as to avoid cancer which is associated with obesity in experimental animals? There are more persuasive reasons.

Jarrett: With regard to height, do we have any reliable information regarding the ideal diet for achieving maximum height? Kiil [1] studied the records of soldiers' heights in Norway from 1830 to 1937. There was an average increase of 0.118 inches per decade from 1830 to 1875, and of 0.236 inches per decade from 1875 to 1937. This was in a fairly homogeneous ethnic group, when breast feeding was, presumably, the norm, and during a century of considerable change in nutritional habits. More anecdotal evidence suggests that other European countries shared in the general increase in stature. It is clear from inspecting medieval suits of armour that the doughty knights of those times were short by contemporary standards. It is commonly believed that nutrition has something to do with these secular changes.

Reference

1. Kiil W (1939) Stature and growth of Norwegian men during the past 200 years. Skr-Nor Vidensk-Akad Oslo 1(6):1–175

Rivers: I do not agree with Naismith's interpretation (pp. 9–12) of the relationship between food intake, activity and height gain. It seems to me that a reduction in activity resulting in a more positive energy balance despite a reduced energy intake could well explain the increase in height observed in the surveys to which he refers.

I agree fully with his suggestion that the old concept of a balanced diet is difficult to define, though I think that it is possible to say something coherent about the concept. I also agree that it may well need revising in the context of an affluent society and that particularly the currently fashionable "healthful diet" may not prove optimal for all sections of the population.

I think, however, that his discussion would be strengthened if he included within it some comments on alcohol, a nutrient which he has omitted to mention. In this he is of course merely doing what we nutritionists are rather prone to do – as for example in Table 1.1, where the distribution of calories between proximate principals is given; neither Naismith nor his source document include reference to alcohol. It is a pity to omit it, since it is probably the one nutrient that we can all agree has a real impact upon health in our society.

Sanders: A discussion of diet needs to include the contribution made by alcohol. Like other aspects of diet, the effects are not clear-cut. Teetotallers aged 34–65 have a higher total mortality rate than moderate drinkers. However, excess alcohol consumption causes cirrhosis of the liver, leads to birth defects, is said to exacerbate gout, increases blood pressure, causes cardiac arrhythmia (holiday heart), contributes towards causing obesity, is a major cause of accidental death and leads to social problems. The pattern of alcohol consumption also determines its effects, bingeing being more harmful than regular consumption. The issue is not whether we should or should not drink, but rather if we do drink, how often and how much we should drink? This is the sort of information people want about diet.

Author's reply: Sanders' catalogue of disaster might indicate that there is no place for alcohol in the balanced diet. Alcohol, like pure sugar confectionery, is, however, metabolised to provide immediate or stored energy (fat). Some individuals may derive a substantial proportion of their energy needs from alcohol. I excluded it from my discussion of the balanced diet simply because it is not an essential nutrient. Vast populations, for religious reasons, do not consume alcohol, and appear to suffer no ill effects. There is clearly no Recommended Daily Allowance. From a nutritional, as well as a clinical viewpoint, the major concern is about the displacement from the diet of foods that contribute useful amounts of the nutrients as well as energy.

Durnin: In general, I found this paper interesting but somehow slightly unsatisfactory in its present context. It does not deal with diets which produce problems: anaemia, which is probably the most common deficiency disease in this country, obesity, diabetes, osteoporosis, etc. There is also no reference made to diet and health for a very important group of the community: the elderly.

Author's reply: I am not aware of specific dietary recommendations for the elderly. A balanced diet for an adult man or woman would no doubt be equally appropriate in old age. There are certainly many problems that may alter nutrient requirements in old age. A very low energy intake resulting from extreme physical inactivity or from illness might lead to an inadequate total intake of protein, vitamins and minerals. Nutrients may be less efficiently absorbed, but the effect would be difficult to quantify. The use of drugs is known to affect the metabolism of several of the nutrients, specifically the vitamins. If those problems are recognised, then, in individual cases, modification of the diet would be justified. Osteoporosis, I am informed (M. Nelson, personal communication), is a disorder caused primarily by a decline in physical activity rather than by a dietary deficiency of calcium, although supplementation of the diet with calcium may retard, but not prevent, the condition.

Jarrett: Naismith's statement on hyperglycaemia and birthweight is too didactic. The relationship between "large for gestational age" (LGA) infants and maternal glycaemia is confounded by maternal age and weight. In a large Australian study [1] hyperglycaemia was more common in the obese but the average birthweight and the frequency of infants weighing more than 4 kg was not related to degree of glycaemia. In the Pima Indians of Arizona there was a significant association between degree of glycaemia and frequency of LGA babies, but this disappeared when controlled for maternal age and obesity [2].

References

1. Calendra C, Abell DA, Beischer NA (1981) Maternal obesity in pregnancy. Obstet Gynecol 57:8–12
2. Pettitt DJ, Knowler WC, Baird R, Bennett PH (1980) Gestational diabetes: infant and maternal complications of pregnancy in relation to third-trimester glucose tolerance in the Pima Indians. Diabetes Care 3:458–464

Rivers: The section on a balanced diet for growth I found most interesting, particularly Naismith's comments on the adverse effects of high-protein feeding in pregnancy, where it appeared to reduce fetal growth, and in the infant, where it accelerated growth. Presumably these effects were manifested as changes in the efficiency of energy utilisation, rather than energy intake? The logic of these observations appears to me to suggest that the optimal diet, at least for the infant, is one in which feed efficiency is not maximal. I am quite willing to accept this.

Dobbing: The suggestion (Naismith's reference 30) that high-protein supplements in pregnancy were associated with a depression of fetal growth, has been the subject of much scepticism over whether the findings justify that conclusion. Many predicted at the time that the statement would be endlessly repeated in later years. Such has proved to be the case, and this is the latest example. The New York study was an unfortunate one in many ways, and I believe it is unwise to take too literal a view of this particular finding.

Southgate: I am not wholly convinced by the argument that subclinical deficiencies do not imply functional impairment; if the biochemical test of nutritional status is functionally based then "subclinical" deficiency is evidence of a functional impairment. The central issue is what criteria should be used to relate morbidity to this functional index of status. (The haemoglobin statement needs to be expanded to have any relevance to the argument.)

Sanders: The values given for mean daily energy intakes in Table 1.1 are unlikely to be reliable estimates. These figures are based on food supply rather than measured intakes and do not take into account differences in the age structure of the populations. For example, in developing countries 40%–50% of the population may be under the age of 15 years. In the Seven Countries Study [1] energy intakes tended to be greater among men from the least affluent countries. It may be wrong, therefore, to conclude that energy intakes are higher in the more affluent countries.

Reference

1. Keys A (1970) Coronary heart disease in seven countries. Circulation 41:1–211

Southgate: In Table 1.1 the order in which the countries are arranged is that of energy value of food moving into consumption per head of population, not daily energy intake. Such estimates are substantially higher than measured intakes. The ranking is arbitrary and does not correspond to measures of affluence or industrialisation. Taking means at intervals is not informative since the groups are entirely arbitrary.

Durnin: I think we should be quite clear that the quantities quoted in Table 1.1 refer to food available for consumption but not actual food intake per head of population. The implications of the information in this table for actual food intakes are based on such imprecise data that I have grave reservations about whether the table has any value for the present purposes.

Curzon: The identification and targeting of at-risk groups may not be impracticable. Dental caries is now, in the United Kingdom, a disease of only 20% of the population. Research in Scandinavia has now produced methods of identifying those children and adults who are at risk of developing dental caries. These people can therefore be targeted for individual dietary counselling and the application of preventive methods.

Jarrett: Naismith's comment about the impracticability of targeting advice may be illustrated by the problems involved in screening for hypercholesterolaemia, as recommended by some. In the first place the accurate measurement of serum cholesterol is technologically difficult, and one estimate is not a good indicator of an individual's usual level. Then, if the 90th centile is taken as that indicating high risk, this means that 10% of the population require dietary advice and, presumably, further monitoring to see whether dietary change is sufficient to reduce the serum cholesterol level. If it is not, then does that mean that drug therapy should be added? Apart from these logistic problems there is the ethical aspect. Is it right to inspire alarm in this large segment of the population, and in effect turn them into patients, with only a limited prospect of reducing their risk of cardiovascular problems?

Curzon: I am concerned about the reference to the diets of the Eskimo. Having lived for some years with the Eskimo in Canada, or Inuit as they should be called, it was my experience that the traditional diet as described by Naismith no longer existed. The use of seal, walrus, bear and caribou is limited and by far and away the food supply is from the Hudson Bay Company stores. As such the diet has a preponderance of flour, which is used in the form of bannock.

Pertinent to the discussion, is that with the Inuit the change to a modern diet from a traditional one has been associated with the continuance of the traditional mode of frequent eating. In the past the use of the foods described by Naismith was variable, as he says, and therefore for most of the year foods were dried and cached for use when game was scarce. Food was then eaten during the times of scarcity as dried meat; this is not easy to consume so the Inuit nibbled it frequently during the day. This habit of nibbling has been carried over to the use of a Western diet. Thus the Inuit might be described as the original "snackers". With a high-carbohydrate diet, based upon starches and sugars, it is not surprising to see in the modern Inuit a very high rate of dental caries.

Southgate: The NACNE discussion paper [1] criticised the use of the term "balanced diet" primarily because the definition of "balanced" was distinctly unclear, and the authors interpreted the derivation of the term as relating to the need to meet the quantitative requirements for minerals and vitamins. Indeed the term "balanced diet" seems to have come into common usage without any formal definition, but my reading of the early literature suggests that "balance" referred to the balance of foods [2]. Thus, an imbalanced diet was a diet limited in respect of the range of foods eaten. Some texts give the impression that balance related to the balance between cations and anions, at a time when the balance between alkali-forming and acid-forming foods was seen as important to health. The most common usage of the term emerges in more recent times as dietary recommendations in terms of constructing the daily diet from foods from food groups [3], although this approach is presented very clearly in Sherman [2].

In present-day use the term "balance" seems to have value in relation to the desirability of balancing the intake of the major nutrients, principally the fats, free sugars and complex carbohydrates. I find this term more explicit than the terms "healthful" or "prudent" [4].

The debate which followed from the McGovern Committee report on Dietary Goals for the United States [5], which has been extended to many countries, and in the United Kingdom culminated in the NACNE discussion paper [1], argues from the proposition that the incidence of many diseases which show a higher incidence in Western, developed and affluent communities is related to dietary intake.

This has been extrapolated into the concept that "health" is a function of the diet and that a change in diet [6] would be associated with a change in health. Since "health" is an integrated concept, involving many attributes besides physical well-being, it is impossible to measure, and the quantitive derivation of the relation with diet is therefore virtually impossible. Disease incidence is, in principle, more easily quantifiable, and it is therefore possible to contemplate deriving a relationship with dietary intake. Dietary goals implicitly embrace the concept that it is possible to define diets that achieve some kind of optimum relationship to disease incidence. Any use of the term "optimal" requires definition, and this is probably one major weakness of national dietary goals, since they do not appear to recognise the fact that optimising diet in respect of a population requires recognition that an optimal diet would vary with developmental age, sex, and level of physical activity. Moreover, optimising in respect of a range of different disease states may produce conflicts.

If, as a working concept, the balanced diet is seen as a diet that provides the "optimal" composition, the central problem is to define what this composition is and which compositional parameters need to be defined. Such a diet must be quantitatively adequate, so that it provides for the quantitative requirements for nutrients, particularly minerals and vitamins. Although experimental data on nutrient requirements are far from adequate, the generalised relationship is believed to be of the form shown in Fig. C.1, so that the balanced diet can be defined in terms of a desirable range of intake. Although excess intakes of water-soluble vitamins above tissue saturation do not usually produce adverse effects, this is not true for the fat-soluble vitamins, where definition of an upper compositional level is necessary. Excessive intakes of many inorganic nutrients can cause inhibition of the absorption of others, so there will be a need for defined ranges of intakes, not merely minimal levels. Furthermore, there is substantive evidence of individual variation in requirements, and the balanced diet should provide nutrients at levels that meet the average requirement with an allowance for the upper range of requirements.

The primary definition of the composition of a diet relates to the balance of the macro nutrients. It is probable that, provided energy needs are met, definition of the diet in a limited range of major components would be adequate. These will describe

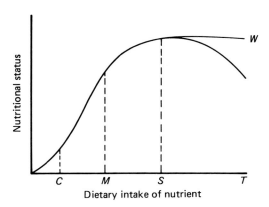

Fig. C.1. Relation between nutritional status and dietary intake. At intakes less than *C* clinical deficiency symptoms occur. Between *C* and *M* status improves rapidly with increasing intake. Between *M* and *S* status responds slowly to increasing intake. At *S* status no longer improves with intake. At *T* toxic effects of excess intake are evident. *W* indicates saturation with water-soluble components and greatly increased urinary secretion.

a "domain" in multidimensional space and in Chap. 7 I examine the evidence for including dietary fibre as one of these compositional dimensions.

References

1. Health Education Council (1983) Proposals for nutrition guidelines for health education in Britain. National Advisory Committee for Nutrition Education, London
2. Sherman HC (1933) Chemistry of food and nutrition, 4th edn. Macmillan, New York
3. DHSS (1978) Eating for health. HMSO, London
4. British Nutrition Foundation (1987) Comment, 8 May
5. Select Committee on Nutrition and Human Needs (1977) Dietary goals for the United States, 2nd edn. US Government Printing Office 052-07004376-8, Washington
6. Gibney MJ (1986) Nutrition, diet and health. Cambridge University Press, Cambridge

Chapter 2

Diet and Obesity

J. V. G. A. Durnin

This paper will not attempt to define the constrictions that "the concept of a balanced diet" might impose upon the general area of "obesity". We will assume that "a balanced diet" would require a provision of energy to the body, as well as of nutrients, which would be appropriate for supplying its needs. We will therefore examine some dietary variations which might influence human energy balance. To undertake this in any comprehensive way requires an examination of the normal composition of the human body, particularly in relation to its fat content, and how, and by how much, the total quantity of body fat may increase.

Introduction

Obesity arises when the intake of energy in the food exceeds the energy expended to the extent that there is a marked increase in the amount of fat present in the body. The imbalance of energy intake and expenditure may happen in several different ways, most of which are hypothetical, since virtually no long-term measurements have ever been done on people leading a free-living, natural and unconstrained existence who have become obese. In theory, energy imbalance leading to obesity might occur over a relatively short time due to gross excesses of intake, or it might arise very gradually. In real life, obesity probably develops by both these pathways, to a variable extent. Many people feel that they put on some extra weight over a fairly short time when their normal routine was disturbed, perhaps when they were on holiday, or if they were working away from home for a time, or if they were perhaps worried or depressed, or, for many women, when they were pregnant and became fatter by more than the physiologically desirable amount. The added weight then seems very difficult to remove, and frequently there are subsequent episodes with more and more superfluous fat accumulating in the body. In all circumstances there has to be a sufficient excess of energy intake to cause the fat deposition. How much energy is in fact involved in this process?

Distinguishing the Physical Factors Involved in Weight Gain

There are only two components of the normal human body which can vary enough to cause an increase in weight, other than very temporarily. These components are fat and muscle. Other tissues may alter, but either minimally or for only very brief periods of time. For example, the skeleton has a relatively small capacity for increasing its mass due to the need to support a greater total body mass, either because of gross obesity or because of prolonged and heavy weight-training. The fluid content of the body can also be augmented by some pathological conditions. Fat and muscle can be very considerably increased and it is quite conceivable that the total body mass could be almost doubled equally well by an increase in either of these tissues. Very heavy, regular and prolonged weight-training can result in very large increases in muscle mass, but clearly this is a rare occurrence in an average population. On the other hand, very big additions to the body mass occur with depressing frequency in the population because of the excess deposition of fat. Indeed, a very large amount of fat in the body will often also be accompanied by an appreciable increase in muscle mass, presumably occasioned by the greater physical effort involved in moving the obese body around.

However, we can reasonably assume that when the body weight increases, in most normal circumstances this is due to an addition of fat to the body. We can also make some simple calculations of how much extra energy is required to deposit a certain amount of fat in the human body. In order to make the calculation reasonably accurate we need to take into account the fact that fat is not laid down in the body simply as fat or chemical lipid but is enclosed in the envelopes of the fat cell membranes, and that these fat cells have fluid spaces around them and that the whole structure is held together by connective tissue. When we get fatter, we are therefore increasing not only the fat but all the other tissues required to contain this extra fat, the whole being "adipose tissue".

The Energy Required to Lay Down "Fat"

Differentiating between "fat" and "adipose tissue" is important because their energy equivalents differ. Fat, or chemical lipid, has an energy content of about 9 kcal (or 38 kJ) per gram, whereas adipose tissue, because it is a mixture of fat, fluid, cell membranes and connective tissue, has an energy equivalent of about 7 kcal/g (29 kJ). Both of these values show a certain amount of variation, depending on the particular site and type of tissue, but the variation is usually relatively small.

It might therefore be supposed, since the body adds weight because of the deposition of adipose tissue, and because adipose tissue has an energy content of 7 kcal/g (29 kJ), that every 7 kcal (29 kJ) of excess energy taken in by the body would result in an extra 1 g of weight being added. This is not quite the case since the mechanical and chemical processes involved in laying down extra stores of adipose tissue are somewhat inefficient, and in fact it requires about an extra 10 kcal (42 kJ) to result in the deposition of 1 g of adipose tissue: in other words, one extra kilogram of weight added to the body needs an excess of 10 000 kcal (42 MJ) of energy intake over expenditure.

The Development of Obesity

With this value in mind, it then becomes possible to hypothesise about how long it takes to gain a given amount of weight. If we envisage a situation where there is an average *excess* of energy intake over energy expenditure of 100 kcal/day (418 kJ), over the space of a year this means 36 500 kcal (153 MJ). Since each 10 000 kcal (42 MJ) excess will result in one extra kilogram of weight, during a year 3.65 kg of weight will be added. In 5 years this is equal to 18 kg or 40 lb.

This is a considerable quantity of mass but the calculation makes an assumption of a regular excess of intake over expenditure of energy and it is doubtful whether this would be a likely occurrence over a period of as long as 5 years. Even as an average, and therefore making the inference that there would be considerable fluctuations from day to day – sometimes the excess being zero and at other times perhaps 400–500 kcal (1700–2100 kJ) – the assumption is still that the weight gain represents a continuing and uninterrupted positive energy imbalance continuing over a 5-year period. This is probably unlikely as a common situation and it might be more plausible to think of the imbalance as progressing intermittently and perhaps taking a much longer time.

Weight gain, from hearsay evidence, seems more often to take place in distinct episodes when perhaps 5 kg or so is added, consternation sets in, and an attempt is made to remove the excess weight. Such attempts are often unsuccessful but probably result in a fairly prolonged period when no further augmentation of weight occurs. The subsequent periodic increases in weight might not commence for several months, and might follow a similar pattern.

Very much more rapid increases in weight would result from much larger excesses. If, for example, a surplus energy intake of 500 kcal/day (2100 kJ) existed, this is equivalent to a 1 kg weight gain every 20 days, or 4.5 kg every 3 months. Of course, 500 kcal (2100 kJ) as a regular average imbalance of energy intake over expenditure appears an inordinately high amount and probably happens only rarely in the development of moderate obesity.

We have not yet defined what we mean by "obesity". This will be discussed in some detail later in this article, but we could immediately make it clear that there is a very great deal of difference between the development of the common condition of "moderate" obesity and the relatively uncommon state of "gross" obesity. Grossly obese people are in an extreme situation which probably involves severe psychological and perhaps also physical aberrations, and the type of diet, *per se*, may have little influence on the development of the condition. Therefore we will not concern ourselves with a consideration of factors related to diet in the causation of *gross* obesity, and we can, reasonably justifiably, ignore circumstances when very large energy intakes, greatly in excess of requirements, are taken over more than a very occasional few days at a time.

There is only a limited amount of published information on the extent and duration of the development of moderate obesity. Very few longitudinal studies have been reported on the changes in the body weight of populations over extended periods of time. Such studies would be very useful in providing some much-needed quantitative information on the actual extent of the excess energy intake and the period of time to which it referred. In a 15-year follow-up of almost 1000 university undergraduates in 1968, Durnin [1] measured the weight changes that had occurred from the time when they had a medical examination at the age of 18–20 years to their existing weight at the age of about 35 years. There were 611 men and 344 women in the group, representing a more or less random sample of the student population of Glasgow University at that time. The mean increase in weight of the men was 8.5 kg and of the women 2.4 kg. About 20% of the men had added more than 14 kg to their initial weight.

These changes in weight can easily be converted into energy terms although the increase in the weight of the women was too small to be of interest in the present context. The mean increase in the men's weight of 8.5 kg, on the other hand, is a significant addition to the fat mass of the body, perhaps not resulting in the group becoming obese but enhancing the chances of future obesity. However, 8.5 kg is equivalent to only 85 000 kcal (356 MJ) which, added over a 15-year period, is equal to 5700 kcal/year (24 MJ) or 16 kcal/day (66 kJ). For the 20% of the men who added more than 14 kg, the equivalent values are 9300 kcal/year (39 MJ) or 25 kcal/day (107 kJ). Even on the assumption that this added weight occurred spasmodically, and perhaps over only 2 or 3 years in all out of the 15 years, this would still have resulted from an excess energy intake of only 125–175 kcal/day (520–730 kJ), which represents a comparatively small quantity of food.

However, even this needs to be set into some sort of context. The importance of an extra 150 kcal (630 kJ) or so per day will obviously be related to its proportion of the normal daily intake. Someone whose normal intake is 1800 kcal/day (7.6 MJ), and one whose normal daily intake is 3200 kcal (13.4 MJ), will notice an extra 150 kcal (630 kJ) rather differently. Similarly, weight gain may also induce very different feelings and have differing effects on individuals some of whom might have an initial body weight of 50 kg and others of 80 kg.

Nevertheless, we can justifiably assume that "moderate" obesity might easily arise from excess intakes, either regular or intermittent, or relatively small amounts of energy per day. The question is whether some specific dietary factor can be important in causing this comparatively small imbalance. What is implied in this question is whether or not the diet needs to be "unbalanced" to result in an excess intake of energy, or whether this excess might still be a possible outcome for someone on a "balanced diet" but with some other complicating variable exerting its effect, such as, for example, physical inactivity.

Variability in Energy Metabolism

However, there is another complicating factor which might make it more difficult for some people to maintain energy balance, and that is related to the variability in metabolic rate which exists between individuals. We are not concerned here with variability due to differing body masses (obviously a man of 90 kg will have, in general, a higher energy expenditure while sitting, walking, or whatever, than a man of 60 kg), but with variability between men, or women, of similar body masses and body composition and engaged in standardised "activities". We have studied this in groups of between 30 and 40 individual men and similar numbers of women [2]. The subjects were selected so that all of those in each group had almost the same body mass (58 ± 2 kg for the women and 68 ± 2 kg for the men) and the same degree of fatness (a range of 3% body fat as measured by densitometry and skinfold thicknesses. Measurements were made of basal metabolic rate (BMR), and of energy expenditure while walking at a fixed rate on a treadmill. There was a standard deviation of about

± 10% in BMR which, translated into the range of energy expended in BMR per day, implies that the 15% of men at the lower end of the range had BMRs which were about 450–500 kcal (1.89–2.10 MJ) less than the BMRs of the 15% at the top end of the range. The equivalent difference in the women was just under 400 kcal/day (1.67 MJ). The energy expended in walking also differed sufficiently (±13%) to result in appreciable variation in the energy expended in walking of similar duration and speed by different individuals.

The fact that these considerable dissimilarities in energy metabolism exist in people who are physically almost identical is clearly likely to impose much greater difficulties on those with a lower metabolic rate in maintaining their energy balance: for similar lifestyles their intake of food will need to be several hundred kilocalories a day less. Such metabolic variability is unlikely to be related to diet.

The Definition and Measurement of Obesity

It is inadequate to discuss the role of any potentially incriminating factor in obesity without attempting some definition of obesity. At present obesity is usually defined on the basis of weight : height (W : H) ratios, and W/H^2 or the Body Mass Index is the popular pseudo-scientific ratio which is most widely accepted. In the very recent Report issued by the British Medical Association Board of Science and Education entitled *Diet, Nutrition and Health* [3] an "acceptable" state is one where W/H^2 equals between 20 and 25. Examples of this range of 20–25 would mean that a woman 5 ft 5 in. tall (1.65 m) ought to weigh between 54 and 68 kg, and a man 5 ft 9 in. (1.74 m) tall between 60 and 75 kg. Obesity is supposed to start when W/H^2 equals 30, or when the woman's weight is 72 kg and the man's 90 kg. What the state is meant to be when W/H^2 lies between 25 and 30 is unclear.

However, life is more complicated than this. The ratio of W/H^2 may be acceptable for population studies when, for example, large groups of people are being contrasted. When this method is applied to individuals, however, it is not appropriate and may indeed be quite misleading. Two people with exactly the same W/H^2 can differ very markedly in their fatness, simply because individuals of the same height may have very different proportions of muscle and various other tissues including the skeleton. Anthropologists interested in somatotyping have known this for many years. This individual variability also becomes obvious when some objective measurement of fatness is made on groups of individuals of the same height and weight. In a recent study on a large number of adult men and women [4] the total sample size of 9000 individuals was large enough to allow groups of about 200 men of the same height and weight to be assessed for fatness by measurement of skinfold thicknesses [5]. The fact that their heights and weights were the same meant, naturally, that they all had the same W/H^2. However, the range of fatness, as estimated by skinfold thicknesses, was very wide and meant that some of the mean were very lean, with 10% of their body weight as fat, and others moderately obese (over 30%). W/H^2 will not reliably discriminate for fatness *for an individual*. It will indicate only relative weight; and it might conceivably be, of course, that "overweight" itself, independently of fatness, is occasionally a medical hazard. However, this would be a confusing element in a discussion of the relationship between a particular foodstuff, such as sugar, and obesity, and presumably sugar or any other foodstuff would be unlikely to influence body weight other than via the fat content of the body.

Classification of Obesity

Obesity and fatness are not synonymous terms. *Obesity* has a definite implication of an undesirable state, either medically, or physiologically, or aesthetically. Frequently these implications have not been properly demonstrated in a controlled scientific fashion. Categories of *fatness*, as the name implies, allow a simple and limited classification of different degrees of fatness in individuals which then permits the analysis of connections between these degrees of fatness and medical risk, or mechanical disadvantage, or aesthetic appeal. The use of the actual value of percentage fatness instead of only the category with its rather wide range is better still because it permits a finer, more precise analysis. Also it provides the opportunity to form quite different classifications if desired.

Fatness, then, requires to be defined if we are to examine any implications of a specific factor on its causation, since otherwise our terms are too uncertain to be meaningful. In terms of the quantity or proportion of fat in the body, which is relatively easily and reasonably accurately measurable by the use of skinfold calipers [6], it is not difficult to define limits of "normal", lean, moderately obese and grossly obese on the basis of the percentage of fat in the total body mass. The acceptance of these limits, with approximately the values suggested in Table 2.1, would probably not arouse too much opposition.

Table 2.1.   A simple classification of fatness

	Young adult men	Young adult women
Lean	⩽10%	⩽20%
"Normal"	11%–20%	21%–30%
Moderate obesity	21%–30%	31%–40%
"Gross" obesity	⩾31%	⩾41%

Values are expressed as percentages of body weight as fat.

Many studies from the United Kingdom and other European, as well as North American, populations have found that an average healthy young adult man has about 15% of his total body weight as fat, the comparable value for women being 25% of the body weight. Lean males such as athletes and very active men would have 10% or less of body weight as fat. The comparable value for lean women would be 20% or less. Moderately obese men and women have 21%–30% and 31%–40% of body weight as fat respectively, and gross obesity exceeds these values. A simple table can be constructed to give quantitative definitions of relative fatness (Table 2.1). These categories are not meant to have rigid boundaries. It is obviously ridiculous to classify a man as "moderately obese" with 30% of his body weight as fat, and "grossly obese" with 31%, especially when no known method of measuring fatness can discriminate to this level. The exact range for "moderate obesity" for women might also be a subject for some discussion and controversy. However, these are minor drawbacks and this classification has the considerable benefit that it depends upon an actual measurement of fatness, and not on a ratio of weight to height. It also allows the percentage fatness to be used as a parameter, not only to allow categorisation.

Age also needs to be taken into consideration in the classification of fatness. As regards children, the adult values remain applicable probably down to the age of 10 years or so [7]. For children below 10 years of age there are no very reliable standards, although W : H ratios are probably even more unreliable than they are for adults. At the other end of the age spectrum, for middle-aged and elderly people there are other factors complicating the formulation of definitions of obesity or categories of fatness, and the above classification of fatness may not be appropriate for most societies in developed countries. The classification suggested here, and most modern indices of desirable weight, make virtually no allowance for an age factor in adults, although this used to be standard practice in the past. It is assumed, in other words, that older men and women should have no greater quantities of fat in their bodies than younger adults.

Some of the data collected in the anthropometric study on 9000 adults in the United Kingdom [4] might justify some modification in this attitude. There is no doubt that, with increasing age, an increasing proportion of the total amount of fat in the body may become internal as opposed to subcutaneous [5,8]. The result of this shift in body fat from the subcutaneous to the internal areas of the body means that any value for skinfold thickness, obtained either by objective measurement or by pinching the skin with the fingers, represents an increasing total amount of fat as age increases. For example, a value of 35mm in a 20-year-old man and in a 45-year-old man represents approximately 15% and 20% fat respectively. Therefore, men over 45 years of age with fat percentages which are average for young men have the superficial appearance of being far leaner than younger individuals.

It becomes questionable, therefore, whether it is realistic to expect the total fat contents of middle-aged and older men to be exactly comparable to those of younger individuals, since this would imply perhaps excessive degrees of leanness, as assessed by physical appearance or by skinfold thickness, in these older individuals. For men in their forties or older there are probably negligible medical reasons for assuming that a mean value of 20% fat, as opposed to an equivalent mean value in young men of 15% fat, represents a serious medical hazard. There are also few well-documented arguments showing any likelihood of a serious mechanical disadvantage, or a negative relationship to "fitness", in having these slightly higher percentages of body fat in middle age. On the other hand, in young men there may well be greater risks attached to these higher mean values, since moderate degrees of obesity acquired between the ages of 20 and 40 years appear to be more detrimental to health than obesity developed in later life [9].

Similar conclusions might reasonably be proposed in the case of middle-aged and older women. As an interim suggestion, the equivalent values for the categories of lean, normal, moderate and gross obesity might be increased uniformly by 5% for men and women over 40 years of age. The maximum values for "normal" men and women over 40 would thus become 25% and 35% respectively, and the other ranges would similarly be increased by 5%.

This is a somewhat arbitrary recommendation, but its usefulness can easily be discovered in practice. It can be supported in at least a semi-plausible way because in the study on 9000 adults [4], 80% of the men over 40 had more than 20% of body weight as fat, and yet were physically active (taking exercise or sport at least twice a week), and almost no men over 40 had 15% or less fat. This does not, of course, mean that these men and women might not have been in a more desirable physical state if their fat contents were similar to those of younger adults. However, until there is better evidence that that statement is usually true, it does not seem very sensible to propose a category of "normal" which is quite appropriate for younger adults but into which only a small minority of healthy, moderately active middle-aged and elderly people fit.

If a measurement of fatness, as opposed to a ratio of weight to height which is obviously potentially erroneous, is to be employed in large-scale field studies, then it has to be obtainable using a relatively simple and quick technique. It has been argued that the measurement of skinfold thicknesses is too difficult and open to too much inter-observer error to allow its use for this purpose. The basis for this negative judgement has little objective justification. Several published papers [e.g. 10,11] have shown the observer error to be small when the measuring technique is standardised [12]. The actual measurement of a skinfold is relatively simple – much simpler usually than taking a valid reading of the blood pressure.

While the use of skinfold thicknesses to determine relative fatness is the simplest, cheapest and most acceptable technique, it is also now possible to do measurements of electrical conductivity on moderate-sized groups of perhaps several hundreds. Newer types of equipment to do this, which is an indirect method of measuring total body water and thus fatness, are also simple to use and are, in general, scientifically acceptable.

Fat Distribution in the Human Body

For many years there has been speculation about the clinical importance not only of obesity but also of the distribution of the excess fat [13]. However, it was only with the use, in this context, of CAT (computerised axial tomography) and NMR (nuclear magnetic resonance) that it became possible to visualise and then actually measure the intra-abdominal and the subcutaneous fat [14]. A somewhat crude anthropometric approximation of this, the waist/hip ratio, i.e. the ratio of the waist to the hip circumference, seemed to demonstrate the possibility of a relationship between this ratio and diseases such as coronary heart disease and diabetes [15,16].

The question of whether there is indeed a close connection between fat distribution, as opposed to general obesity, and disease is at a very elementary stage of resolution, and the best way of measuring this distribution by simple field techniques is still also a matter for debate. Nevertheless, it is a very interesting development in the whole area of the medical importance of obesity, and it may well cause us to reassess some of our rather crude assumptions.

Several field studies are presently being conducted with the main object of assessing the variability of different populations in relation to the waist/hip ratio and of investigating the connection between this ratio and hormone levels (e.g. free and total testosterone). The assumption at present is that obesity with a preponderance of a male distribution of fat (a high waist/hip ratio) is more dangerous than a typical feminine distribution with a low waist/hip ratio. However, some preliminary results from a comparison of middle-aged women in four different European countries (Italy, Sweden, Holland and Poland) indicate appreciable differences in this ratio between the women from the different countries. Clearly, much research will need to be done on this problem before definitive conclusions can be reached. In any case, it appears improbable (though not impossible) that diet may have an influence on the relative distribution of the adipose tissue.

The Relationship Between a Foodstuff (Sugar) and Obesity

A diet can be unbalanced in respect of the various nutrients. For example, there is the somewhat uncommon situation of a deficiency of protein in the context of adequate energy, or alternatively an excess of fat, or inadequate minerals or vitamins. None of these, with the exception of excess fat, is directly related to obesity nor will it necessarily lead to obesity. Excess fat will predispose to obesity only if there is also an excess of total energy.

An unbalanced diet will therefore be associated with obesity in situations where, independently of the actual amount of energy in the diet, the intake is in excess of the expenditure. This may occur through influences operating mainly either on the "intake" side of the equation or on the "expenditure" side. That is, excess intake may be present because certain foodstuffs in the diet are so attractive that they encourage overeating. However, it is also possible to have an excess intake as a result of very low expenditure of energy due to low levels of physical activity. If physical activity is virtually non-existent, it may become too difficult in the long term to restrict the dietary intake to quantities that just balance expenditure, and eventually obesity results. This latter state is almost certainly very common in our sort of society, where work and transport are such that only small amounts of physical activity are absolutely necessary, and where temptations to be inactive, such as sitting watching television for large parts of the non-working day, are commonplace. Studies on adolescents [17,18] have clearly shown very large reductions in their mean daily energy intake in the past 50 years, where there has been no complicating factor of changing work activity because of increasing mechanisation.

However, this contributing factor to obesity, probably by far the most important single influence, is not strictly related to the concept of a "balanced diet" and will not be discussed further. As far as diet is concerned, it is necessary to examine the likelihood that single foodstuffs, or combinations of foodstuffs, could predispose to the intake of excess energy, and thus lead to obesity.

The foodstuff most commonly suggested as fitting this role is sugar and sugar-containing foods. Sugar is popularly supposed to be consumed in large quantities by the majority of the population of the United Kingdom, is commonly regarded as a superfluous item of diet by many so-called expert nutritionists and dietitians, and may well be the single most frequent cause of an "unbalanced diet". It may be useful to consider whether or not obesity can be linked to the intake of sugar by individuals.

Sugar is, of course, an energy-rich substance. Its energy content is about 400 kcal/ 100 g (1.71 MJ). However, there are many foods of similar energy content, some of them containing a certain amount of sugar. Examples are most biscuits and cakes, sugared breakfast cereals (e.g. Cornflakes, Rice Crispies), almost all cheeses, cheese omelette, grilled chops, fried sausages, sausage rolls and fried whitebait. A multitude of foods contain more than half the energy, per 100 g, of sugar: bread, fried and scrambled eggs, boiled beef, lean roast beef, grilled steak, lean boiled ham, roast pork, raw herring, fried sole and plaice, canned sardines, fried mushrooms or onions. currants and raisins, dates, figs. And several foods contain very much more energy than sugar: butter and margarine, fried bacon, potato crisps, many nuts, chocolates, shortbread.

One might speculate that it would be more palatable to eat much larger quantities of many of these foods, such as bread, biscuits, breakfast cereals, meats, eggs, cheeses, fried fish, than to eat the equivalent quantity of sugar. So the argument becomes very complex. It is really not possible to come to any conclusion about the role of sugar, or indeed of any other foodstuff, in the causation of obesity on the basis of its energy content or on a comparison with other foods of similar or greater or lesser energy. The excess energy required in the long term to produce obesity is small enough for almost any food to be incriminated. If an obese individual has a particular liking for sweet food, or fatty food, or peaches, or apples, or almost anything, it is possible to argue that the reason for the obesity is that the predilection for the specific foodstuff meant that more food energy was taken in the diet than was absolutely required for energy balance, and that this more or less consistent excess energy intake, perhaps of very small quantity, eventually led to obesity.

Lay people would probably reject such a theory with scorn, the implication appearing to be that foods which are very tasty and attractive might make one obese, and the corollary being that one is more likely to avoid obesity if the food one eats is not particularly appetising.

While it would also be generally accepted that many people do indeed have "a sweet tooth", or enjoy fried food, particularly potato chips (or "fries" or "pommes frites" or "crisps"), these likings are not necessarily associated with obesity. From the strictly scientific viewpoint, and taking cognisance of all of the problems involved in validating a connection between particular foodstuffs and obesity, the development of obesity cannot sensibly be blamed on individual foods which might be part of a person's average diet. The suggestion can be based on the likelihood of the total intake of energy tending to become excessive due specifically to the presence of certain foods in the diet. But proving such a proposition requires either exceptionally clear-cut distinctions between different diets or exceptionally well-controlled studies on, probably, fairly large populations. It also implies not only the requirement to measure fatness in the population being studied, but also to have longitudinal data available so that it can be shown either that the presence of a specific foodstuff, such as sugar, leads to progressive fatness, with sugar being the isolated variable, or else that a reduction in sugar or its withdrawal from the diet leads to a progressive loss of weight which is maintained over a sufficiently prolonged period. To suggest that sugar is implicated in the causation of obesity on the basis of a short-term (12 days) reduction in energy intake in a small number of men when foods containing sucrose were replaced by aspartame-containing foods [19] is not convincing-enough evidence that the same situation would apply on a wider scale and over a prolonged period.

There are cross-sectional studies which show that some populations, whose diet contains significantly less sugar than others, are also less obese. But these cannot be interpreted in any simplified manner. For the inferences which can be drawn from such a study to be persuasive, all of the other variables which might also affect fatness, such as the level of energy intakes, the way of life of the populations, their levels of physical activity, probably also their attitudes to fatness, would need to have been carefully controlled. There are many distinct factors which might be the principal reason for the obesity, and isolating one of these is extremely difficult. Another problem in cross-sectional studies relating sugar intake to obesity is the possibility, sometimes mentioned but extremely difficult to interpret accurately, that a lower sugar intake in obese individuals might indicate only a changed pattern of eating resulting from the obesity. The obese person might, in the past, have had a higher sugar intake and might now be trying to lose weight by reducing the amount of sugar in the diet. Quantifying this type of situation is virtually impossible.

However, in many areas related to the development of obesity the impossibility in practice of controlling all the variables perfectly makes it unrealistic to expect absolutely incontrovertible scientific evidence proving the proposition. On the other hand, there ought to be a reasonable volume of good evidence pointing fairly conclusively in one direction. The example which has been chosen to analyse the probability that an unbalanced diet can lead to obesity – that is that foods containing sugar, and/or sugar itself, are the incriminating agents – appears, at least superficially, to be the one most easy to prove. The evidence against sugar in relation to its involvement in the causation of obesity needs to be examined carefully.

A Review of the Literature

Several reports have been published during the past few years on "healthy diets", and they include sections on obesity. In the United Kingdom the most recent document is the Report of the Board of Science and Education of the British Medical Association on *Diet, Nutrition and Health* [3]. There is no doubt about their view of sugar. Sugar is regarded not only as a foodstuff the consumption of which should be reduced for non-specific reasons, but a foodstuff which is specifically related to obesity. For weight reduction, "foods rich in fat and sugar need to be restricted on a long term basis". It should be noted that the discussion about whether or not a reduction in sugar intake will be useful in the *treatment* of obesity is a completely different topic from whether or not sugar is an important element in the *causation* of obesity. Obviously, many items of food are capable of being withdrawn from an average diet and, if they are not replaced by something else, energy intake will fall and weight should be lost. The easiest foods to include in this category would be either very energy-dense foods, particularly fatty foods, or foods the withdrawal of which would cause a minimum of psychological disturbance to the obese person. Such foods would not necessarily have any direct connection with obesity, but simply be relevant to a reduced energy intake, and they are not strictly within the current context. This discussion will therefore concentrate on whether or not sugar is an important contributory factor to the development of obesity.

Another document of some obvious interest is the Report on Obesity of the Royal College of Physicians of London [20], which is an extensive and excellent review of many aspects of obesity. However, even though it is most comprehensive it hardly mentions sugar, or any other specific foodstuff, other than to state in a very general way that obese people should be encouraged to reduce fat and sugar in their diet.

Another Report, entitled *Research on Obesity*, by a UK Department of Health and Social Security/Medical Research Council group [21], examined many areas particularly requiring research. No mention was made of sugar intake as a topic worth considering.

In the United States a conference on "Obesity in Pespective" was held at the Fogarty International Centre at the National Institutes of Health in Bethesda. This also was a wide-ranging examination of obesity as a public health problem, and the two-volume proceedings [22] cover most aspects of the problem. However, apart from some brief studies on various taste preferences of obese and non-obese subjects which were not related to total energy intake, sugar is barely mentioned.

A bibliography [23] of what must be most of the published papers on obesity between 1964 and 1973 gives one pertinent reference [24]. A group of 415 businessmen completed a questionnaire about sugar intake and this was related to their relative weight. In fact there was an inverse relationship between the sugar eaten and "fatness", the fatter men having a lower intake. Many of them did state, though, that at the time of the questionnaire they were restricting their intake of sugar. There was also an interesting positive relationship between sugar intake and exercise levels, the more active men apparently eating more sugar. More recent symposia, conferences and review articles are equally unhelpful in providing hard information on this relationship. Apart from these Reports, reviews, and published proceedings of symposia and congresses, there is a very limited number of relevant original publications. At the metabolic level, Swaminathan et al. [25] showed no difference in the thermic effect of giving 400 kcal (1.67 MJ) of sugar to lean and obese subjects, thus suggesting that sugar intake should be unaffected by metabolic influences. This finding is also supported by Welle and Campbell [26] in a similar study.

With regard to actual intake of sugar in the diet, several papers have reported either no difference in sugar intake between obese and lean individuals, or sometimes a negative relationship. Three examples, typical of these papers, are given below:

1. A study by Garn et al. [27] found that intakes of sugar foods were no higher among obese than among lean persons in a group of 4907 adolescents in the USA Ten-State Nutrition Survey.

2. Examination of data from the nationwide survey in the United States of 972 children aged between 5 and 18 found no general relation between eating patterns and obesity (assessed by weight/height ratios). However, the authors [28] felt that more homogeneous samples were required before definitive conclusions could be reached.

3. A study in Wales on 493 men aged 45–59 [29], where food intake was measured by the 7-day weighted individual inventory method, found that sugar intake was negatively associated with the body mass index (W/H^2).

However, an individual's actual present-day intakes of sugar have limited validity in assessing whether or not sugar is a significant factor in *causing* obesity. Evidence of a different and superficially more persuasive kind could be obtained from psychological studies of food preferences in obese and non-obese people. It if could be shown that obese people have a marked preference for sweet foods, compared with the non-obese, then it might appear that this could induce them to eat more than they absolutely require for energy balance.

It has been argued earlier in this article that preferences for any foodstuff are physiologically unlikely to result in excess energy intake unless they upset the regulation of energy balance; that is, unless they influence our appetite-controlling system in such a way that it is unable to fulfil its normal function of informing the higher centres in the brain that enough food has been ingested. There is no good evidence that this occurs either with sugar or sugar containing foods, or with fats. Nevertheless, it is still interesting to see whether some food preferences differentiate obese and non-obese people.

An excellent review by Grinker [30] effectively seems to demolish what she calls "one of the more prevalent myths about factors associated with the genesis of obesity, that obese individuals have a 'sweet tooth'". She concludes her review by saying that "obese individuals are not more sensitive to sweet taste" and that their "taste preferences for sweet are equivalent to or lower than those of normal weight individuals". Another psychologist, Rodin [31], has similarly concluded that moderately overweight individuals do not display marked discrimination of sweet taste from normal weight subjects, nor do they show a greater preference for sweets than normal. An investigation of taste preferences for various fat–sugar mixtures by Drewnowski et al. [32] on normal-weight and obese subjects found that normal-weight subjects optimally preferred mixtures containing 20% fat and less than 10% sugar, whereas obese subjects preferred high fat mixes (more than 34% fat) which contained less than 5% sugar.

Low-energy foods, or low sucrose diets, must have been tested in relation to weight reduction on innumerable occasions. Their efficacy has certainly not been demonstrated [33]. Weight loss is unrelated to cutting down on sugar, whereas cutting down on fat or increasing activity levels are positively correlated to weight reduction [34].

Finally, two quotations from some of the individual contributions in a very recent book on *Sweetness* [35] make it very difficult to believe in any close connection between sugar and obesity.

Food selection does relate to satiety in a manner that may be relevant to weight control, but it has nothing specific to do with sweetness . . . if sugars contribute to obesity the problem is likely to be "inefficient" satiation rather than high palatability. [36]

. . . there is little direct evidence that the diet of obese individuals is rich in sweetened foods. On the contrary, epidemiological surveys of different populations have repeatedly observed an inverse relationship between reported sugar consumption and the degree of overweight [28,38] . . . No behavioural observations are at present available that might distinguish between different classes of obesity on the basis of taste responsiveness profiles or the patterns of food selection. [39,37]

General Conclusions

The analysis of such evidence as is available, the most pertinent of which has been examined here, is that a specific foodstuff, sugar (or sugar-containing foods), even though it *might* usefully be reduced when an obese person is attempting to lose weight, appears to play no important role in the generation of obesity. At the least, it is unlikely that it does play such a role, and proving it has such enormous practical difficulties that it becomes almost impossible.

The lack of balance in the diet which eventually leads to obesity must therefore be sought in ways other than through the influence of some particular foodstuff. One of these might, of course, be eating habits. Perhaps people who become obese eat fewer main meals, or eat more snacks, than the non-obese. Some animal experiments have suggested this [40], but little evidence has ever been found of a similar situation in man. It is tempting to think that frequent "snackers", people who seem continually to be munching potato crisps or eating chocolate bars, are the ones who become fat. This has not been shown to be generally true. It is in any case improbable. Some recent studies on energy intake on over 100 women whose intakes were measured on several consecutive days and repeated on many different occasions (6 to 16 times) throughout a year [41] have shown such very large variability from day to day (several hundred kilocalories) and from period to period, that the operation of a single dietary influence causing them to overeat is difficult to comprehend.

The solution must be searched for from a different angle. The excess energy intake which causes the imbalance in the diet might persuasively be attributed to an energy expenditure which is too low to be continually satisfied by a comparatively low intake. As has been argued earlier, the fact that such a large percentage of the whole population in many developed countries appears to be overweight might easily reflect the progressive diminution in the quantity of necessary physical activity in daily life, which leads to an energy expenditure of relatively low levels for many people. The required energy intake to balance this involves eating quantities of food which are, from time to time, too small to satisfy our appetites. Occasional overeating will eventually lead to obesity. It is not the diet which is unbalanced, it is the energy output.

References

1. Durnin JVGA (1968) The change in body weight of a young adult human population after an interval of 15 years. J Physiol (Lond) 198:22
2. Durnin JVGA (1983) The variability of dietary energy. In: Kevaney J (ed) Energy balance in human nutrition. Royal Irish Academy, Dublin, pp 13–23
3. British Medical Association (1986) Diet, nutrition and health. Report of the Board of Science and Education. British Medical Association, London
4. Durnin JVGA, McKay FC, Webster CI (1985) A new method of assessing fatness and desirable weight, for use in the Armed Services. Report to Ministry of Defence, London
5. Durnin JVGA, Womersley J (1974) Body fat assessed from total body density and its estimation from skinfold thickness: measurements on 481 men and women aged from 16 to 72 years. Br J Nutr 32:77–97
6. Norgan NG (1986) Human body composition and fat distribution. Euro-Nut report 8. Agricultural University, Wageningen
7. Brook CGD (1971) Determination of body composition of children from skinfold measurements. Arch Dis Child 46:182–184
8. Skerlj B, Brozek J, Hunt EE (1953) Subcutaneous fat and age changes in body build and body form in women. Am J Phys Anthrop 11:577–600
9. Van Itallie TB (1979) Obesity, adverse effects on health and longevity. Am J Clin Nutr 32:2723–2733
10. Womersley J, Durnin JVGA (1973) An experimental study on variability of measurements of skinfold thickness on young adults. Hum Biol 45:281–292
11. Burkinshaw L, Jones PRM, Krupowicz DW (1973) Observer error in skinfold thickness measurements. Hum Biol 45:273–279
12. Weiner JS, Lourie JA (1981) Practical human biology. Academic Press, London
13. Vague J, Combes R, Tramoni M, Angeletti S, Rubin P (1979) The diabetogenic adipose mass. In: Mancini M, Lewis B, Contaldo F (eds) Medical complications of obesity. Academic Press, London, pp 45–58
14. Heymsfield SB (1986) Human body composition: analysis by computerized axial tomography and nuclear magnetic resonance. In: Norgan NG (ed) Human body composition and fat distribution. Euro-Nut report 8. Agricultural University, Wageningen, pp 105–112
15. Sjostrom L, Krist H, Lapidus L, Bergtsson C, Tylen U (1986) Weight–height indices and adipose tissue distribution: measurements and health consequences. In: Norgan NG (ed) Human body composition and fat distribution. Euro-Nut report 8. Agricultural University, Wageningen, pp 189–198
16. Bjorntorp P (1986) Fat patterning and disease: a review. In: Norgan NG (ed) Human body composition and fat distribution. Euro-Nut report 8. Agricultural University, Wageningen, pp 201–209
17. Widdowson EM (1947) A study of individual children's diets. Medical Research Council Special Report Series 257. HMSO, London
18. Durnin JVGA, Lonergan ME, Good J, Ewan A (1974) A cross-sectional nutritional and anthropometric study, with an interval of 7 years, on 611 young adolescent schoolchildren. Br J Nutr 32:169–179
19. Porikos KP, Hesser MF, Van Itallie TB (1982) Caloric regulation in normal weight men maintained on a palatable diet of conventional foods. Physiol Behav 29:293–300
20. Royal College of Physicians (1983) Obesity: a report. J R Coll Physicians Lond 17:1–58
21. DHSS (1976) Research on obesity: a report of the DHSS/MRC Group. HMSO, London
22. Bray GA (1975) Obesity in perspective. DHEW publication NIH 75–708. Parts I and II. DHEW, Washington
23. Whelan H, Silverstone T (1974) Obesity: a bibliography. Information Retrieval Ltd, London
24. Richardson JF (1972) The sugar intake of businessmen and its inverse relationship with relative weight. Br J Nutr 27:449–460
25. Swaminathan R, King RFGJ, Holmfield J, Siwek RA, Baker M, Wales JK (1985) Thermic effect of feeding carbohydrate, fat, protein and mixed meal in lean and obese subjects. Am J Clin Nutr 42:177–181

26. Welle SL, Campbell RG (1983) Normal thermic effect of glucose in obese women. Am J Clin Nutr 37:87–92
27. Garn SM, Solomon SA, Cole PE (1980) Sugar-food intake of obese and lean adolescents. Ecol Food Nutr 9:219–222
28. Morgan KJ, Johnson SR, Stampley GL (1983) Children's frequency of eating, total sugar intake and weight/height stature. Nutr Res 3:635–652
29. Fehily Am, Philipps KM, Yarnell JWG (1984) Diet, smoking, social class, and body mass index in the Caerphilly heart disease study. Am J Clin Nutr 40:827–833
30. Grinker J (1978) Obesity and sweet taste. Am J Clin Nutr 31:1078–1087
31. Rodin J (1977) Implications of responsiveness to sweet taste for obesity. In: Weiffenbach J (ed) Taste and development: the genesis of sweet preference. DHEW publication 77–1068. DHEW, Bethesda
32. Drewnowski A, Brunzell JD, Sande K, Iverius PH, Greenwood MRC (1985) Sweet tooth reconsidered: taste responsiveness in human obesity. Physiol Behav 35:617–622
33. Finer N (1985) Sugar substitutes in the treatment of obesity and diabetes mellitus. Clin Nutr 4:207–214
34. Lewis VJ, Booth DA (1985) Causal influences within an individual's dieting thoughts, feelings and behaviour. In: Leitzman C, Diehl JM (eds) Measurement and determinants of food habits and food preferences. Euro-Nut report 5. Agricultural University, Wageningen
35. Dobbing J (1987) Sweetness. Springer-Verlag, London Berlin Heidelberg New York
36. Booth DA, Conner MT, Marie S (1987) Sweetness and food selection: measurement of "sweetness" effect on acceptance. In: Dobbing J (ed) Sweetness. Springer-Verlag, London Berlin Heidelberg New York
37. Drewnowski A (1987) Sweetness and obesity. In: Dobbing J (ed) Sweetness. Springer-Verlag, London Berlin Heidelberg New York
38. Keen H, Thomas BJ, Jarrett RJ, Fuller JH (1979) Nutrient intake, adiposity and diabetes in man. Br Med J i:655–658
39. Drewnowski A (1985) Food perceptions and preferences of obese adults: a multidimensional approach. Int J Obes 9:201–212
40. Fabry P (1969) Feeding pattern and nutritional adaptations. Butterworth, London
41. Durnin JVGA, McKillop FM, Grant S, Fitzgerald G (1985) Is nutritional status endangered by virtually no extra intake during pregnancy? Lancet 823–825

Commentary

Rivers: Durnin points out that in fattening humans an additional 10 kcal must be consumed to gain 1 g adipose tissue of energy value 7 kcal. If this is taken as the partial energy cost of fattening it would place humans at the lower end of observed values, with a partial efficiency of fattening of only 70%. In animal experiments [1] such values are observed only on low fat diets where fat is synthesised from carbohydrate. On diets with fat levels like those in the United Kingdom a partial efficiency of fattening of about 90% seems to me more likely, since endogenous fatty acid synthesis will be low, and dietary fatty acids will be incorporated into adipose tissue triglycerides. Presumably the reason for the low partial efficiencies observed by Durnin is that some protein is gained as well as fat. If only 8% of the metabolisable energy is retained as protein with an energy value of 5.6 kcal/g, and a partial efficiency of synthesis of 35%, and the remainder retained as fat with an efficiency of 90%, the overall efficiency of energy gain will be about 75%. This seems to me more likely than the concept that significant amounts of mechanical work are involved.

Reference

1. Bernier JF, Calvert CC, Famula TR, Baldwin RL (1987) Energetic efficiency of protein and fat deposition in mice with a major gene for rapid postweaning gain. J Nutr 117:539–548

Naismith: One of the most important advances in the study of obesity in recent years has been the clarification of the role of heredity as a major determinant of all degrees of adiposity, from extreme thinness to extreme fatness [1]. This aspect of obesity was rightly neglected in the present context. Nevertheless it raises the question of how the genetic difference between the lean and the obese manifests itself. Confining ourselves to possible answers that fall within a discussion of "the balanced diet", could it be that the overweight and obese are simply unable to match a "natural" intake with a low level of energy expenditure, as suggested by Durnin, or do they choose a diet differing from that of the lean, which encourages weight gain? The former proposition, if it rests solely on energetics, requires that the obese, on average, expend less energy than do the lean, and so fall below a critical level at which the maintenance of a balance between intake and expenditure is no longer possible, or that the lean have a more flexible response to variations in energy intake. This difference is worth exploring further.

The notion that certain qualities of the diet induce obesity (e.g. high energy density, high content of sucrose) is widely believed, but rarely examined critically as Durnin has done. The meaning of "energy density" has been discussed in my own paper. It is worth noting that an increase in the proportion of sucrose in the diet would either have no effect on energy density (if it replaced starch or protein) or would reduce energy density if it replaced fat. It is frequently argued that one should eat less sugar and more unrefined carbohydrate (i.e. starch plus associated fibre). This would lead to a small reduction in energy density, but given the large day-to-day fluctuations in normal energy intake reported by Durnin, it seems extremely unlikely that the resulting fall in energy intake would not be compensated. A large increase in fibre intake (by other means) might well prove more successful in depressing energy intake, but this could be achieved even without a reduction in sugar consumption. The two forms of carbohydrate ("refined" and "unrefined") are, for the most part, not interchangeable in the diet. Sucrose is used in food manufacturing (domestic and commercial) for two reasons – its taste and its physico-chemical properties (adding to sour fruits and bitter beverages, making jam, cakes, biscuits, confectionery) – neither of which is shared with starch, with or without associated fibre.

Durnin, to my satisfaction, in his review of the published human studies, has dismissed the idea that sucrose encourages the obese (but not the lean) to eat too much food. We must therefore seek some hedonistic property other than sweetness to explain the hyperphagia. In some animal studies [e.g. 2,3] it has been claimed that dietary sucrose does indeed increase total energy intake and promote excessive fat deposition. We have recently repeated these experiments (Naismith and Maitland-Smith, unpublished results) using the same strain of rat and a similar, more elaborate experimental design. We found no evidence that rats offered sucrose either as solid sugar or in solution (32% aqueous sugar solution) in addition to an adequate diet, or as a constituent of the diet (20%), had a higher energy intake or a higher proportion of body fat. Energy derived from sucrose was substituted precisely for energy from the basic diet, thus, at the same time lowering energy density. We did note, however, that rats, like man, display great variability in their liking for sugar.

References

1. Stunkard AJ, Sorensen TIA, Hanis C et al. (1986) An adoption study of human obesity. N Eng J Med 314:193–198

2. Kanerak RB, Orthen-Gambill N (1982) Differential effects of sucrose, fructose and glucose on carbohydrate induced obesity in rats. J Nutr 112:1546–1554
3. Granneman JG, Wade GN (1983) Effects of sucrose over feeding on brown adipose tissue lipogenesis and lipoprotein lipase activity in rats. Metabolism 32:202–207

Jarrett: Durnin's comment about "gross obesity" (a state which is not defined until later) is very much *ex cathedra*. If, for the sake of argument, one takes a lower limit of BMI of 35 to segregate the grossly obese, then what evidence is there of severe psychological aberrations in such people? In some yes, but the majority? In any case in many societies being "grossly obese" is acceptable, even desirable.

Durnin tabulates definitions of fatness based upon fat as a proportion of body weight but, despite the disclaimer about the categories not having rigid boundaries, there is no justification provided for the boundaries. Although I do not agree with them [1] the BMI categories quoted do have *some* observational validity. For observational studies there is no need to have *categories* of fatness. The value can be used as a continuous variable and adjusted for age, sex etc.

Reference

1. Jarrett RJ (1986) Is there an ideal body weight? Br Med J 293:493–495

Author's reply: I agree that my statements about "gross obesity" are perhaps contentious and not precisely validated. The point I was trying to make is, nevertheless, one which I think has much importance and relevance to the present topic. That is, obesity is very often treated as if it were a homogeneous entity and, in my view, this leads to considerable confusion. While there is obviously no absolutely clear-cut division in "obesity", there are the great majority of moderately obese people and a small minority of grossly obese people who have, I consider, a completely different degree of problems.

The grossly obese would be people with a BMI of 40+, and their health, physiological and aesthetic problems are of altogether a different degree of magnitude, and probably of aetiology, to those of the moderately obese person.

In relation to Jarrett's comment on the "observational validity" of the BMI categories, this is true only in a limited way and for some disease conditions. The "safe" range of BMI extends much further than 25. It may go up to 32 in women, for example, and 20 is at a comparatively "unsafe" level.

Sanders: The discussion is preoccupied with refuting the association between sugar intake and obesity. I agree with Durnin's conclusion, and on a physiological basis there is no good reason why sugar should be regarded as more fattening than cooked starches. Between-country comparisons can be made to show an association between percentage energy derived from fat and prevalence of obesity. James [1] has argued that fat may be more fattening than carbohydrate on the basis of limited metabolic studies. It was argued that the theoretical cost of fat storage from dietary cabohydrate is greater than that from dietary fat. Adipose tissue fatty acid composition tends to reflect dietary fat intake, which suggests that relatively little carbohydrate is converted to fat and deposited in adipose tissue. This also implies that dietary carbohydrate is the preferred energy substrate. What evidence is there that decreasing the proportion of energy derived from fat decreases the risk of obesity? Are diets high in carbohydrates less fattening than those high in fat?

Reference

1. James WPT (1985) Is there a thermogenic abnormality in obesity. In: Garrow JS, Halliday D (eds) Substrate and energy metabolism. John Libbey, London, pp 108–118

Macdonald: I am a little confused about the contribution of physical activity to the maintenance of body weight. Some authors feel that the greatest contribution to 24-hour energy output is the basal metabolic rate and superimposed on this is the relatively small proportion of energy output due to physical work. The impression I get from this contribution seems to be the reverse.

Author's reply: While BMR does indeed contribute most to energy output (for a 70-kg sedentary man, perhaps 1600 kcal out of a total of 2500 kcal/day), the influence of physical activity may be very important, although small. A diet of 2500 kcal may not represent a great deal of food and many 70-kg men might have difficulty in restricting themselves to this quantity. Expending an extra 200 or 300 kcal/day in physical activity might easily make a difference to maintaining energy balance.

Southgate: The conclusion that it is impossible to link sucrose or any other component, or a specific foodstuff, with the development of obesity is consistent with my analysis of the general relation between diet and disease. In fact the formal analysis indicates that it is unreasonable to expect such a relationship to emerge.

One important attribute of a balanced diet emerges from this paper: the need to balance energy intake with energy expenditure or vice versa.

The possible role of dietary composition as a determinant of food choice, in its widest sense, might be subject to experimental analysis, but the level of dietary control achievable in free-living populations would not be adequate to measure energy intakes with the required level or precision. Nor indeed, can the conventional use of energy conversion factors or metabolisable energy values from food tables achieve this required level.

The case against sugar or any other energy-yielding component is therefore unproven. However, there is suggestive evidence that the rates of entry of nutrients into the body and metabolic pathways determine metabolic efficiency, and the balance between carbohydrate energy entering as glucose or short-chain fatty acids may have metabolic effects that alter lipid deposition.

Chapter 3

Diabetes Mellitus: Consideration of Diet in Aetiology and Management

R. J. Jarrett

A World Health Organisation Study Group [1] has recently proposed a simple classi-fication of diabetes mellitus into three principal groups (Table 3.1) which differ in their clinical, epidemiological and aetiological features. While this classification must be regarded as provisional, given the remaining uncertainties concerning aetiology, it will be used as the basis for the following discussion. Furthermore, the symposium topic, the balanced diet, will be discussed under two headings: aetiology and treat-ment respectively.

Table. 3.1. Clinical classes of diabetes mellitus

Insulin-dependent diabetes mellitus (IDDM)
Non-insulin-dependent diabetes mellitus (NIDDM)
Malnutrition-related diabetes mellitus (MRDM)
Other types of diabetes associated with certain
   conditions and syndromes

Diet and the Aetiology of Diabetes

Insulin-Dependent Diabetes Mellitus (IDDM)

IDDM is predominantly a disorder presenting in children, adolescents and young adults (hence the previous description "juvenile-onset"), with peak incidence in early adolescence. Incidence rates vary widely, with a more than twenty-fold difference between countries of high incidence (e.g. Finland) and those of low incidence (e.g. Japan) (see Table 3.2). In several countries, such as Finland and Scotland, incidence rates have increased substantially over the past decade, although in others, such as the United States, rates have been stable. In those countries where studies have been performed there are several consistent features: peak incidence in adolescence, association with certain HLA loci on chromosome 6, presence of circulating islet cell antibodies at or near diagnosis, disorders of cellular immunity and, in a limited

Table 3.2.   Some estimates of incidence of young-onset IDDM

Place	Years	Age group	Rate per 1000 Male	Rate per 1000 Female	Total
Europe					
Denmark	1970–76	0–14	14.5	13.4	14.0
Norway	1973–77	0–14	18.8	16.4	17.6
Sweden	1977–80	0–14	21.7	19.8	20.8
Finland	1970–79	0–14	29.7	27.3	28.6
Scotland	1968–76	0–18	14.4	13.2	13.8
France	1975	0–14	–	–	3.7
North America					
Montreal, Canada	1971–77	0–16	8.6	9.0	8.8
Allegheny County, USA	1965–76	0–20	16.02	14.79	(white)
			10.10	11.06	(non-white)
Oceania					
New Zealand	1968–72	0–19	–	–	10.4
Asia					
Japan	1980	0–18	–	–	0.54

number of twin studies, a 50% concordance rate. There are also associations with autoimmune disorders affecting the thyroid and adrenal glands, and current theories hypothesise that IDDM is an autoimmune disorder triggered by unknown environmental factors, of which viruses have received the most attention [2].

There is very little evidence to suggest that dietary factors might be included amongst the environmental determinants. A study in Iceland [3] provided circumstantial evidence that heavy consumption of food rich in nitrites in Christmas/New Year festivities led to an increased incidence of IDDM in children with a birth date in September, though this was confined to male infants. Nevertheless, there are certain substances, such as streptozotocin and PNU (*N*-3-pyridylmethyl-*N*-*p*-nitrophenol), which are relatively specific, islet B cell poisons [4], so it remains possible, though purely speculative, that some cases of IDDM might be provoked by dietary constitutents in predisposed individuals.

Non-Insulin-Dependent Diabetes Mellitus (NIDDM)

NIDDM is the predominant variety of diabetes in all countries. As with IDDM (Table 3.3) there are large variations in prevalence between populations. In Europid* populations incidence is directly related to age, with peak rates in the seventh or eighth decade. In some Third World or developing countries, where the incidence of NIDDM has increased enormously since World War II, NIDDM occurs commonly at younger ages and the relationship with age is more complex and may well be complicated by cohort effects. In all populations there is a relationship between degree of

*Freedman [5] debates the use of the word "Caucasian" to denote "white Europeans" and finds it, together with several alternative terms, to be unsatisfactory, indeed inappropriate. The term "Europid" was introduced by Peters [6] and is en suite with negrid, mongolid, australid, etc. Etymologically it is more correct than Europoid (cf. Caucasoid, negroid, etc.) for the suffix "-oid" implies a resemblance to some definitive concept whereas the suffix "-id(e)" implies "of the family of".

Table 3.3. Age-standardised diabetes prevalence rates per 1000 population[a] for the Pacific Region (1975–1981)

Geo-ethnic group	No. studied (≥ 20 yrs)	Diabetes prevalence/1000
Micronesians		
Nauru	456	303
Polynesians		
Tuvalu	397	39
W. Samoa (r)[b]	745	27
W. Samoa (u)	744	70
Melanesians		
Loyalty	535	20
New Caledonia	172	15
Fiji (r)	477	18
Fiji (u)	861	69
New Guinea (u)	184	154
Indians		
Fiji (r)	452	133
Fiji (u)	848	148

Source: Zimmet [15].

[a] Age standardised to Western Samoa Census (1976).

[b] r, rural; u, urban.

obesity and incidence/prevalence of NIDDM. More recently attention has shifted to consideration of the distribution as well as the amount of fat and several studies have demonstrated a stronger relationship between incidence or prevalence of NIDDM and central distribution of fat than with Body Mass Index (BMI) or other indices of overall obesity [7].

A strong genetic contribution to the aetiology of NIDDM is suggested by a twin study in the United Kingdom where concordance rates for NIDDM in identical twins approached 100% [8]. In the remarkable Pima Indians of Arizona, who hold the unenviable world record for high diabetes prevalence [9], an incidence study showed an exponential relationship between NIDDM incidence and BMI in those with one or both parents having NIDDM, but only a small positive relationship when neither parent had NIDDM – despite the fact that half the subjects had a BMI exceeding 30 kg/m^2 [10].

It is this variety of diabetes in which a dietary aetiology has long been implicated. Thus West [11] quotes Hindu physicians of the sixth century as attributing diabetes "to overindulgence in rich foods". Thomas Willis, the seventeenth-century English physician in his aptly titled monograph *Of the diabetes or pissing evil* [12], stated: "the diabetes was a disease so rare among the ancients that many physicians made no mention of it; and Galen knew only two sick of it. But in our age, given to good fellowship and guzzling down chiefly unalloyed wine, we meet with examples and instances enough, I may say daily, of this disease".

If one accepts the considerable evidence that excess fat tissue is one of the major determinants of NIDDM then those old and anecdotal comments make sense in that fat will only accumulate when caloric intake exceeds output, though this is not necessarily due to "overindulgence in rich foods" or to gluttony in the Lucullian sense of the word (after Licinius Lucullus, a wealthy Roman, famous for the luxury of his banquets).

Attempts have been made to incriminate more specific items of the diet. These include excess carbohydrate and/or sucrose, excess fat and reduced consumption of fibre-rich starchy foods. The literature up to the mid-1970s is extensively reviewed by West [11] and little new evidence has been adduced since then. Apart from the anecdotal, most of the evidence for the involvement of any of these items is based upon inter-population comparisons or within-population comparisons across time. With few exceptions, potentially confounding variables are not considered, nor the fragility of some of the variables, such as mortality data for NIDDM [13].

Epidemiological studies in the Pacific Region have documented the changes associated with the evolution from a subsistence to a cash economy [14,15]. Several diseases or disorders are associated with such change – obesity, hypertension, diabetes, dental caries, coronary artery disease, hyperuricaemia and gout – along with numerous dietary changes. In the subsistence economy the typical diet is characterised by the consumption of local fruits and vegetables (usually high in fibre and carbohydrate), supplemented by fish. This has changed to a diet characterised by consumption of rice, flour and sugar with more total calories, fat and salt. These changes include all of those suggested to be individually responsible for determining an increased incidence of diabetes. Of course there are many other lifestyle changes, of which a reduction in physical activity may be particularly relevant to the risks of obesity and diabetes.

Another example of the protective effect of traditional lifestyle may be adduced from the studies of Japanese in Hiroshima compared with migrants to Hawaii [16]. In the latter island the prevalence of diabetes was approximately twice that in Hiroshima and obesity much more frequent. The total caloric intake was similar but the Hawaiian Japanese consumed approximately twice as much fat, one third less complex carbohydrate and almost three times as much simple carbohydrate. They also had a much higher frequency of coronary heart disease. Again, the comparison is potentially confounded by many other differences in lifestyle.

In both of the examples quoted, it is worth noting that the cumulative effect of the lifestyle differences includes an increase in the frequency of obesity, which, in the context of NIDDM, if not of other disorders, may be most relevant.

Prospective studies are generally reckoned the most powerful epidemiological method for determining risk factors. Only two have reported the relationship between diet and subsequent development of diabetes. In an Israeli study of 10 000 male civil servants, Medalie et al. [17] carried out an extensive dietary study at the baseline examination and then followed the group for 5 years. There are no significant associations in univariate analysis between either total energy intake or any other dietary variable and the incidence of NIDDM. In the Pima Indians [18] diet was assessed by a 24-hour recall method in 277 female subjects aged 25–44 years. Eighty-seven developed NIDDM over the follow-up period and they had a significantly higher baseline carbohydrate and starch consumption. There were no significant differences in other constituents – fat (saturated/unsaturated), protein (animal/ vegetable) – or in total calories.

Two case-control studies have been reported, both from the United Kingdom. Himsworth [19] concluded that, before the onset of symptoms, diabetics consumed diets of higher calorie content, in particular of higher fat content. Baird [20] also observed that diabetics consumed more total calories than their non-diabetic siblings but that the percentage of energy derived from each of the constituents was the same in each group. By contrast, cross-sectional studies relating diet and glucose tolerance have demonstrated better glucose tolerance in high calorie consumers [21].

There is therefore no consistent evidence to support the thesis that the constitution of the diet modifies the risk of developing NIDDM. However, given the relative crudity and lack of reliability in individual estimates of dietary intake, particularly in epidemiological studies (cf. the weak or absent correlations of fat intake and coronary heart disease within populations), the notion cannot be discarded. Nevertheless, the most reasonable interpretation of currently available data is that the risk of NIDDM would be minimised by a diet which avoids the accumulation of body fat. Other risks under discussion at this symposium, in particular atherosclerosis, are probably more relevant to the balance of the diet.

Malnutrition-Related Diabetes Mellitus (MRDM)

The WHO Study Group [1] has recommended the new term, malnutrition-related diabetes mellitus (MRDM), to include previous descriptive terms such as tropical diabetes, pancreatic diabetes, pancreatogenic diabetes, endocrine pancreatic syndrome, phasic insulin dependence and ketosis-resistant diabetes of the young.

The WHO Study Group has also stated that there are two major subtypes of MRDM: (1) fibrocalculous pancreatic diabetes (FCPD) and (2) protein-deficient pancreatic diabetes (PDPD).

Fibrocalculous Pancreatic Diabetes (FCPD)

The first clear description of this syndrome was provided by Zuidema from Indonesia [22]. He described seven young patients with pancreatic calcification, of whom six had diabetes. Of these, three also had parotid gland enlargement, a feature often associated with malnutrition.

Since Zuidema's classic paper, similar cases have been reported from Bangladesh, Brazil, India, Jamaica, Madagascar, Nigeria, Sri Lanka, Thailand, Uganda, Zaire and Zambia. The pathology comprises diffuse pancreatic fibrosis with stones in the main and subsidiary pancreatic ducts. There is usually a male predominance (up to 3 : 1), onset is usually below 30 years of age and a history of recurrent abdominal pain is common. At presentation the patients are usually underweight, often grossly so, hyperglycaemia is moderate to severe, and most patients require insulin, often in high dosage, to control the blood glucose. Ketoacidosis may occur, but appears to be relatively uncommon.

Unlike the chronic pancreatitis familiar to physicians in industrialised countries, associated gall bladder disease and/or alcoholism are rare in FCPD. Furthermore, although deficiencies in exocrine function may be demonstrable, they are not often severe.

Protein-Deficient Pancreatic Diabetes (PDPD)

Hugh-Jones [23] reported from Jamaica a consecutive series of 215 diabetics of whom 13 had an unusual variety characterised by a requirement for high doses of insulin associated with resistance to ketosis. The subjects were mainly lean and with onset between the ages of 10 and 40 years. Hugh-Jones suggested the description J-type for this variant of the diabetic syndrome. Subsequently, similar cases have been reported from Bangladesh, Brunei, Fiji, Ghana, India, Indonesia, Kenya, Malawi, Malaysia, Nigeria, Papua New Guinea, South Africa, Uganda, Tanzania and Zaire. There is no consistent sex difference in reported cases and, by definition, pancreatic calcification is absent. As with FCPD, there are often clinical indications of present or past malnutrition.

Pathogenesis of Malnutrition-related Diabetes Mellitus

Although in his original report Zuidema [22] implicated malnutrition in the pathogenesis of FCPD, the distribution internationally of reported cases does not coincide with that of the predominant forms of malnutrition, kwashiorkor and marasmus. Clinical observations [24] suggested an association between pancreatic disease and the consumption of cassava, and McMillan and Geevarghese [25] subsequently reported a positive geographical association between cassava production/consumption and the incidence of malnutrition-related diabetes.

A possible biochemical/toxicological explanation for the association lies in the fact that cassava is potentially a major source of dietary cyanide. Cassava root contains several cyanogenic glycosides, principally linamarin, which liberate hydrocyanic acid under hydrolysis. Cyanide can be detoxified by several biochemical reactions, mainly by sulphur-containing amino acids. The principal end-product is thiocyanate, which explains the association between cassava consumption and goitre. Cassava is also a very poor source of protein and particularly of sulphur-containing amino acids. Apart from cassava, other staple foods commonly used in tropical countries, such as yams, peas, beans, sorghum and millet, are also potential sources of cyanide.

These observations led to the hypothesis that cyanide consumption, in association with a low protein diet, in some way causes damage to the pancreas. Conversely, when protein intake is adequate, thiocyanate detoxification may lead to goitre formation. McMillan and Geevarghese [25] reported some experimental work in rats in which they were able to produce temporary hyperglycaemia, but not permanent diabetes, by chronic cyanide ingestion.

However, so far as human malnutrition-related diabetes is concerned, the cyanide hypothesis still requires confirmation. The epidemiological association between cassava consumption and MRDM is by no means uniform. Thus in India, in the state of Kerala there is a strong correlation between the incidence of MRDM, in particular FCPD, and the consumption of cassava. However, in Madras and in other parts of India, MRDM occurs in populations which rarely consume cassava.

At present there are no good data concerning the incidence of MRDM in any population, and understanding of the possible role of dietary factors in the genesis of the disorder would be helped by some systematic epidemiological enquiries. Attention should be paid to the possibility that toxins other than cyanide may be potential pancreatic pathogens, whether as normal constituents of food or as contaminants (cf. aflatoxin and liver cancer).

Diet and the Treatment of Diabetes

Before 1921 the only therapy for diabetes was by dietary manipulation, and some degree of success could be achieved, even in classical diabetics, by gross restriction of carbohydrate [26]. The diets used necessarily contained a large proportion of fat in order to provide sufficient calories. This practice influenced diabetic diets for several decades, even though the availability of insulin had completely altered the situation.

In 1924 Joslin wrote "the diet in health is made up chiefly of carbohydrate; the diet in diabetes is made up chiefly of fat" [27], but by 1928 he was questioning "can it be that the prevalence of arteriosclerosis in diabetes is to be attributed to the high fat diets we have prescribed and more especially to these diets having been rich in cholesterol? I suspect this may be the case. At any rate it is reasonable to maintain the cholesterol in the blood of our patients at a normal level and that I shall strive to do" [28]. Nevertheless, in 1975, a survey of dietary prescriptions used in British diabetic clinics revealed that most prescriptions in use involved substantial reduction in carbohydrate as the cornerstone of dietary treatment advice [29]. Whether diabetics actually followed this advice is another matter [30].

Despite several publications reporting little or no change in blood glucose control or in insulin requirement with more liberal quantities of dietary carbohydrate, "official" advice remained conservative until the 1970s. Advice then changed for a number of reasons.

Concern with the higher risk of atherosclerosis in diabetics led researchers to evaluate the effect of relatively high carbohydrate, low fat regimens. Thus Stone and Connor [31] compared the then standard American Diabetes Association (ADA) diet (41% carbohydrate; 42% fat – about half saturated; cholesterol content 800–1000 mg) in 25 patients with an experimental diet (64% carbohydrate; 20% fat – about one fifth saturated; cholesterol content 100 mg) in 31 patents, who included 6 subjects with persistent hyperlipaemia on the ADA diet. Over a 12-month follow-up insulin requirements remained stable in both groups, but in the experimental group there were substantial falls in both cholesterol and triglyceride levels. Several other groups [32] reported qualitatively similar results; quantitative differences may, in part, have been due to the nature of the fat in the control diets rather than the amount and also to the nature of the carbohydrate sources.

In the 1970s Trowell [33] proposed, on the basis of diverse observations, that a low fibre intake might predispose to the development of NIDDM. Whether true or not, his writings probably stimulated research on the role of fibre in the management of diabetes. A number of short-term studies [34,35] have claimed that changing to a high-fibre diet improves glycaemic control (or allows reduction in hypoglycaemic therapy) and leads to a reduction in cholesterol and triglyceride levels. In most such studies the trial design has been of poor quality, but that of Rivellese et al. [36] can be quoted with approval, except for its short timescale. In this study 8 diabetics (4 IDDM, 4 NIDDM) ate three different diets for 10-day periods. Diet A comprised 53% carbohydrate and 16 g fibre, Diet B 53% carbohydrate and 54 g fibre, and Diet C 42% carbohydrate and 20 g fibre. Each diet had an identical ratio of polyunsaturated to saturated fat and the source of fibre comprised foods normally eaten in Italy. Diet A was given first, then B or C in random order. Both 2-hour post-prandial and mean daily glucose levels were significantly lower after diet B, as were total and low density lipoprotein (LDL) cholesterol levels. Total and very low density lipoprotein (VLDL) triglyceride levels after diet B were significantly lower than after diet A but were not different from those after diet C. High density lipoprotein (HDL) cholesterol concentration was not affected by diet B but was significantly higher after diet C.

Mann and colleagues have carried out slightly longer studies using a cross-over design and 6-week study periods. In the first study a conventional diet was compared with one high in cereals and vegetables (carbohydrate 59% with 44 g fibre) [37,38]. In patients with IDDM and NIDDM the experimental diet resulted in significantly lower fasting and pre-prandial, but not post-prandial, blood glucose levels and glycated haemoglobin levels. There were also significant reductions in total and LDL cholesterol. Fasting triglyceride levels did not change significantly. Following up the result of other studies on the effects of guar and pectin in reducing post-prandial glycaemia [39], a second study used an experimental diet which included substantial quantities of cooked dried beans as readily available sources with physiological effects resembling those of guar and pectin [40,41]. This experimental diet had a substantially greater effect on glycaemia, including post-prandial blood glucose levels. It also reduced total and LDL cholesterol levels without any change in triglyceride, and reduced levels of several coagulation factors shown in a prospective study to be predictive of coronary heart disease [42,43].

This study, together with the very short-term experiments, provides circumstantial evidence to support the current "official" recommendations for the use of high carbohydrate, high fibre diets in diabetic patients. However, a number of questions remain. Would the putative beneficial effects upon risk factors for vascular disease persist in the long term and would there be real benefit in prevention of vascular disease? The practical problems of implementing the advice are exemplified by the longer-term study of McCulloch et al. [44] in which the experimenters managed to persuade their subjects to consume only 45.4% of energy as carbohydrate and to raise their average fibre intake to only 31.8 g per day. Even in the Oxford study, only a minority of subjects persisted with the high fibre intake after the end of the experimental period and in one study 2 of 15 patients recruited could not tolerate the high fibre diet because they found it unpalatable. As the regime required beans to be eaten at two meals each day there would also be practical problems in terms of meal preparation, particularly if other family members wanted something entirely different.

A reasonable conclusion from the experimental studies is that there is no good reason to restrict carbohydrate specifically in diets of diabetics. There is less certainty about the merits or demerits of various carbohydrate sources – high fibre/low fibre or simple/complex carbohydrate molecules. Many are currently examining the so-called glycaemic index of individual foods and of mixed meals and whether or not sucrose might be included in a diet prescription [45,46]. While no doubt of scientific interest, it is difficult to believe that their outcome will be recommendations to individual patients. Furthermore although dietary practices are becoming much more open to outside influences, the local culture remains an important determinant of both choice and availability of foods, and any recommendations must take this into account if they are to be followed.

The discussion hitherto has related to diabetics in general, but certain high-risk groups merit special attention. Thus patients with hyperlipaemia would have a greater incentive to observe a high carbohydrate/low fat regimen. Dodson and colleagues [47,48] in short-term (3-month) studies with moderately hypertensive subjects achieved impressive reductions in blood pressure with low sodium [47] and combined high fibre, low fat and moderate sodium restriction [48] respectively. In insulin-dependent diabetics with proteinuria the rate of decline of glomerular filtration rate was substantially diminished when the diet was changed to one low in protein [49].

Conclusion

In attempting to recommend a balanced diet for diabetics one faces the same problem as recommending one for the generality of mankind, namely deciding what the objective is. If it is to diminish morbidity and delay mortality then in a population of diabetics under medical management therapeutic strategy might reasonably be related to individual risk. Thus if weight/plasma lipids/blood pressure are normal then should one worry unduly about total calories/fat intake/salt respectively? Or, as the majority of diabetics in the United Kingdom are above age 65 years [50], should they be subject to the same dietary prescription as the younger minority? These questions are similar to those raised in the debate about the relative merits of the population and high-risk strategies for prevention of ischaemic heart disease [51,52]. As an epidemiologist I lean to the former, but as a clinician to the latter.

References

1. Diabetes mellitus: report of a WHO study group (1985). World Health Organisation, Geneva (Tech Rep Ser 727)
2. Spencer KM, Cudworth AG (1983) The aetiology of insulin dependent diabetes mellitus. In: Mann JI et al. (eds) Diabetes in epidemiological perspective. Churchill Livingstone, Edinburgh, pp 99–121
3. Helgason T, Jonasson MR (1981) Evidence for a food additive as a cause of ketosis-prone diabetes. Lancet II:716–720
4. Anon (1979) Pesticidal diabetes. Br Med J ii:292–293
5. Freedman BJ (1984) Caucasian. Br Med J 288:696–698
6. Peters HB (1937) Die Wissenschaftlichen Nomen der menschlichen Körperformgruppen. Z Rassemkunde 6:211–241
7. Ohlson L-O, Larson B, Svärdsudd K et al. (1985) The influence of body fat distribution on the incidence of diabetes mellitus: 13.5 years of follow-up of the participants in the study of men born in 1913. Diabetes 34:1055–1058
8. Barnett AH, Leslie RDG, Pyke DA (1982) Twin studies in non-insulin-dependent diabetes. In: Köbberling J, Tattersall R (eds) The genetics of diabetes mellitus. Academic Press, London pp 225–232
9. Bennett PH, Rushforth NB, Miller M, Le Compte PM (1976) Epidemiologic studies of diabetes in the Pima Indians. Recent Prog Horm Res 32:333–376
10. Knowler WC, Pettit DJ, Savage PJ, Bennett PH (1981) Diabetes incidence in Pima Indians: contributions of obesity and parental diabetes. Am J Epidemiol 113:144–156
11. West KM (1978) Epidemiology of diabetes and its vascular lesions. Elsevier, New York
12. Willis T (1679) Of the diabetes or Pissing Evil. Pharmaceutice Rationalis. T Dring, C Harper, J Leight, London, chapt 3, part 1
13. Fuller JH, Elford J, Goldblatt P, Adelstein AM (1983) Diabetes mortality: new light on an underestimated public health problem. Diabetologia 24:336–341
14. Prior IAM, Rose BS, Harvey HPB, Davidson F (1966) Hyperuricaemia, gout and diabetic abnormality in Polynesian people. Lancet I:333–338
15. Zimmet P (1982) Type 2 (non-insulin-dependent) diabetes – an epidemiological overview. Diabetologia 22:399–411
16. Kawate R, Yamakido M, Nishimoto Y, Bennett PH, Hamman RF, Knowler WC (1979) Diabetes mellitus and its vascular complications in Japanese migrants on the island of Hawaii. Diabetes Care 2:161–170
17. Medalie JH, Papier C, Herman JB et al. (1974) Diabetes mellitus among 10 000 adult men. I. Five year incidence and associated variables. Isr J Med Sci 10:681–697
18. Bennett PH, Knowler WC, Baird HR, Butler WJ, Pettitt DJ, Reid JM (1984) Diet and development

of non-insulin-dependent diabetes mellitus: an epidemiological perspective. In: Pozza G et al. (eds) Diet, diabetes, and atherosclerosis. Raven Press, New York, pp 109–119

19. Himsworth HP, Marshall EM (1935) The diet of diabetics prior to the onset of disease. Clin Sci 2:95–115

20. Baird JD (1972) Diet and the development of clinical diabetes. Acta Diabetol Lat 9(suppl 1):621–637

21. Keen H, Thomas BJ, Jarrett RJ, Fuller JH (1978) Nutritional factors in diabetes mellitus. In: Yudkin J (ed) Diet of man; needs and wants. Applied Science Publishers, London, pp 89–108

22. Zuidema PJ (1955) Calcification and cirrhosis of the pancreas in patients with deficient nutrition. Doc Med Geog Trop 7:229–251

23. Hugh-Jones P (1955) Diabetes in Jamaica. Lancet II:891–897

24. Pitchumoni CS (1973) Pancreas in primary malnutrition disorders. Am J Clin Nutr 26:374–379

25. McMillan DE, Geevarghese PJ (1979) Dietary cyanide and tropical malnutrition diabetes. Diabetes Care 2:202–208

26. Allen FM (1924) The dietetic management of diabetes. Am J Med Sci 167:554–570

27. Joslin EP (1924) A diabetes manual for the mutual use of doctor and patient. Lea and Febiger, Philadelphia

28. Joslin EP (1928) A diabetes manual for the mutual use of doctor and patient. Lea and Febiger, Philadelphia

29. Truswell AS, Thomas BJ, Brown AM (1975) Survey of dietary policy and management in British diabetic clinics. Br Med J iv:7–11

30 West KM (1973) Diet therapy of diabetes: an analysis of failure. Ann Intern Med 79:425–434

31. Stone DB, Connor WE (1963) The prolonged effects of a low cholesterol, high carbohydrate diet upon the serum lipids in diabetic patients. Diabetes 12:127–132

32. Van Eck WF (1959) The effect of a low fat diet on the serum lipids in diabetes and its significance in diabetic retinopathy. Am J Med 27:196–211

33. Trowell HC (1976) Definition of dietary fibre and hypothesis that it is a protective factor in certain diseases. Am J Clin Nutr 29:417–427

34. Kiehm TG, Anderson JW, Ward K (1976) Beneficial effects of a high carbohydrate, high fiber diet on hyperglycaemic diabetic men. Am J Clin Nutr 29:895–899

35. Anderson JW, Kyllen W (1979) High carbohydrate, high fiber diets for insulin treated men with diabetes mellitus. Am J Clin Nutr 2:2312–2321

36. Rivellese A, Riccardi G, Giacco A et al. (1980) Effect on dietary fibre on glucose control and serum lipoproteins in diabetic patients. Lancet II:447–452

37. Simpson RW, Mann JI, Eaton J, Carter RD, Hockaday TDR (1979) High carbohydrate diets and insulin-dependent diabetes. Br Med J ii:523–525

38. Simpson RW, Mann JI, Eaton J, Moore RA, Carter R, Hockaday TDR (1979) Improved glucose control in maturity-onset diabetes treated with high-carbohydrate modified fat diet. Br Med J i:1753–1756

39. Jenkins DJA, Wolever TMS, Haworth R, Leeds AR, Hockaday TDR (1976) Guar gum in diabetes. Lancet II:1086–1087

40. Simpson HCR, Simpson RW, Lousley S et al. (1981) A high carbohydrate–leguminous fibre diet improves all aspects of diabetic control. Lancet I:1–5

41. Lousley SE, Jones DB, Slaughter P, Carter RD, Jelfs R, Mann JI (1984) High carbohydrate–high fibre diets in poorly controlled diabetes. Diabetic Med 1:21–25

42. Meade TW, Mellows S, Brozovic M et al (1986) Haemostatic function and ischaemic heart disease: principal results of the Northwick Park heart study. Lancet II:533–537

43. Simpson HCR, Mann JI, Chakrabarti R et al. (1982) Effect of high fibre diet on haemostatic variables in diabetes. Br Med J 284:1608

44. McCulloch DK, Mitchell RD, Ambler J, Tattersall RB (1985) A prospective comparison of "conventional" and high carbohydrate/high fibre/low fat diets in adults with established Type 1 (insulin-dependent) diabetes. Diabetologia 28:208–212

45. Jenkins DJA, Wolever TMS, Jenkins AL, Josse RG, Wong GS (1984) The glycaemic response to carbohydrate foods. Lancet II:388–391

46. Mann JI (1987) Simple sugars and diabetes. Diabetic Med 4:135–139

47. Dodson PM, Beevers M, Hallworth R, Webberley MJ, Fletcher RF, Taylor KG (1987) Sodium and blood pressure in the hypertensive type II diabetic: randomised blind controlled and cross-over studies of moderate sodium restriction. Proc Nutr Soc 46:22 (abstract)

48. Dodson PM, Pacy PJ, Bal P, Kubicki AJ, Fletcher RF, Taylor KG (1984) A controlled trial of a high fibre, low fat, and low sodium diet for mild hypertension in Type 2 (non-insulin dependent) diabetic patients. Diabetologia 27:522–526

49. Bending JJ, Dodds R, Keen H, Viberti GC (1986) Lowering protein intake and the progression of diabetic renal failure. Diabetologia 29:516 (abstract)
50. Gatling W, Houston AC, Hill RD (1985) The prevalence of diabetes mellitus in a typical English community. J R Coll Physicians Lond 19:248–250
51. Rose G (1981) Strategy of prevention: lessons from cardiovascular disease. Br Med J 282:1847–1851
52. Oliver MF (1983) Should we not forget about mass control of coronary risk factors? Lancet II:37–38

Commentary

Rivers: Knowing how difficult it is to measure food intake accurately, and how labile food habits appear to be, I find it difficult to accept studies where a single dietary measurement is taken as a measure of the diet consumed over the next 5 years. I am not surprised when such studies fail to show a relationship with disease, such as in the Israeli study by Medalie et al.; and I am astounded when associations are reported, as with the study on Pima Indians. I concede that the existence of a relationship means that the diet questionnaire measured something that had predictive value of risk, but I wonder if it is necessarily nutrient intake? It is not impossible, for example, that the response is a measure of personality and that this is the predictor of risk.

Curzon: In this paper the conclusion is proposed that there is no good reason to restrict carbohydrate specifically in diabetics. However, if this is so the use of refined carbohydrates should not be frequent because of the risk of dental caries. Being medically compromised and at a greater risk of infection it is important that diabetics do not develop dental caries.

Author's reply: Diabetics are in practice advised to avoid sucrose, though there is recent evidence that sucrose as part of a meal may be no more hyperglycaemic than other carbohydrate sources. In diabetic children sweets and confectionery are often allowed, with the advice to include them with meals as part of the carbohydrate allowance.

Southgate: It is worth commenting on the poor quality of the dietary intake data, particularly those in prospective studies. Many authors ignore the effect of the observation on food choice, either as recorded or as reported by the subject; and in the context of today's exposure to media views on good nutrition, many respondents report a better diet than that actually consumed, frequently using a misguided notion of "better".

MacGregor: From a common-sense point of view, if obesity is closely related to non-insulin-dependent diabetes mellitus, is it likely that there is some difference in diet to account for the obesity, or is the diabetes itself causing the obesity?

Curzon: Our own work on dental disease and diabetes has shown that, once the patient has been stabilised, there is no difference in dental disease patterns between diabetic and control children. It is worthy of note that these children, as part of the stabilisation, eat a rigorously controlled diet. It could therefore be argued that they eat a balanced diet.

Sanders: Jarrett discusses the relationship between diabetes and cardiovascular diseases and appears to attribute the high prevalence of congestive heart disease in diabetics to high plasma cholesterol and triglyceride concentrations. High plasma lipid concentrations are not a feature of insulin-dependent diabetics (IDDM). Moreover, insulin-dependent diabetics have very different lipoprotein profiles compared with non-insulin-dependent diabetics (NIDDM). For example, high density lipoprotein (HDL) cholesterol concentrations tend to be high in IDDM but low in NIDDM, and total cholesterol concentrations tend to be normal in IDDM but may be elevated in NIDDM. Microvascular disease is a characteristic of diabetes mellitus. This appears to be more strongly related to haemostatic variables than to plasma lipid concentrations. Several studies have shown high rates of platelet turnover in diabetics as well as elevated levels of clotting factors. The higher risk of congestive heart disease in IDDM may well be related to haemostatic factors rather than plasma lipid concentrations.

With regard to NIDDM, hypertriglyceridaemia is common and this is associated with raised levels of clotting factors. Restriction of energy intake in these subjects leads to amelioration of these factors and improved diabetic control. The conclusion that the risk of NIDDM would be minimised by a diet which avoids the accumulation of body fat relates to the total energy consumed rather than the proportion of calories derived from fat or carbohydrate. I believe most studies show that diabetic control is improved when energy intake is restricted, regardless of whether the calories are provided by carbohydrate or fat. Similarly, there appears to be little difference in control when sugars are replaced by cooked starches. A view held by some diabetologists is that frequent consumption of small amounts of carbohydrate is preferable to the consumption of two of three large meals. This advice is in conflict with the evidence concerning the prevention of dental caries, which suggests that frequency of consumption of carbohydrate is the main factor involved. Perhaps this is an example of the difficulties in defining a balanced diet.

Chapter 4

Dietary Carbohydrate and Dental Caries

M. E. J. Curzon

Introduction

In a balanced diet those components which may affect dental caries will be used judiciously, so that any enhancement of the dental caries process is controlled. It is now well known that not all individuals are susceptible to dental decay to the same degree, so the use of dietary carbohydrate will not bring about the same prevalence of decay in all people. Any fermentable carbohydrate used frequently will encourage dental caries in some caries-prone subjects; however, other individuals will experience no decay despite the use of highly cariogenic foods.

There is growing concern with dietary effects on tooth decay, as part of a much larger interest in health. A nutritional survey in 1985 showed that almost two thirds of British housewives were making a deliberate attempt to improve the family diet [1]. In Switzerland the designation "safe for teeth" has been officially approved for confectionery and some oral proprietary medicines found to have passed a cariogenicity test. These tests arose because of a need to advise the public as to which foods should be used in a balanced diet. The controversy that still occurs within the dental research community arises because some scientists believe that sucrose is the only food responsible for dental caries, the "arch enemy of teeth" [2], whereas others, while agreeing that sucrose is a major cause, believe that other dietary carbohydrate may be involved to a greater or lesser degree [3]. It is the reasons for this disagreement that are to be reviewed.

Evidence from Human Studies

Studies on human populations have been of two types: assessment of dental caries in natural populations which have changed their dietary patterns and, more recently, surveys by dietary analysis which are then related to caries prevalence or incidence. Intervention studies have been very rare, owing to the difficulty of controlling the diet of a group of people without infringing their rights and lifestyles.

Historically dental caries in man has been low, although all skull material of whatever period shows some degree of decay [4]. In populations which have rapidly changed their diet in the past century, such as the Canadian Eskimo, dental caries has increased with the change to a high carbohydrate diet [5]. The evidence from the Keewatin Eskimo showed that, while sucrose use was considerable, there had also been a simultaneously dramatic increase in the use of white flour.

Other natural experiments have occurred where a major change has come about in the diet of a group of people. The effect of wartime dietary restrictions on dental caries during World War II, was one such natural intervention which has been reported by a number of authors [6–8]. In several countries sugar consumption was reduced in favour of an increase in the use of potatoes, other vegetables and oils. In all the reviews of these wartime changes it has been shown that the drop in dental caries was due to a reduction in the use of sucrose [7–9]. On the other hand an improvement in the general nutrition of the child population may have influenced the development of the teeth and thus account for the lag period between dietary changes and the drop in dental caries [10]. During the war period so many dietary changes occurred, including the extraction rate of flour, frequency of eating and other aspects of lifestyles, that it is not possible to identify which effect was actually responsible for the decline in caries.

The amount of sugar in the diet consumed per capita has been related by Sreebny [11] to the average level of dental caries in a number of countries. He claimed that countries with low consumptions of sucrose had a low prevalence of caries. This approach depended entirely on data collected from a multitude of sources of doubtful comparability. It also relied on sucrose data based on production and not consumption.

Experiments where the quantities of sugar consumed have been artificially changed are rare, because of the difficulty of carrying out such research ethically. The classic study at Vipeholm [12] was completed before strict rules on the conduct of human research came into force. Nevertheless this report on the cariogenicity of foods forms the basis for much of our knowledge.

Vipeholm Study

The Vipeholm study provided substantial evidence for a link between diet and caries experience. Inmates of a Swedish institute for the mentally retarded were fed several types of carbohydrates – sugar, toffee, bread and chocolate – at various frequencies between or during meals. The incidence of dental decay over a 3-year period was monitored and related to the use of the various carbohydrate regimens. Those patients receiving the highest levels of sucrose, 330 g/day with their meals, experienced minimal increases in caries. However, patients eating smaller quantities of sucrose between meals developed high levels of caries. Even when the sucrose was used in different forms, such as caramels or toffees, the main determinant of decay was the frequency of intake rather than its quantity. Traditionally this study has been quoted to prove that sucrose causes caries [9]. Yet a critical look at the Vipeholm study shows that the main finding is that frequency of intake of whatever carbohydrate used determined the incidence of dental caries [10].

Hopewood House Study

An Australian businessman attributed his own good health to a natural diet devoid of any refined or processed carbohydrates. In Hopewood House in New South Wales (Australia), the home he founded for 80 young orphan children aged 7 to 14 years of age, the diet was therefore essentially vegetarian and low in sugars. After a 10-year period the children of Hopewood House had a mean DMFT score (decayed, missing, filled teeth) of 1.6 compared with 10.7 in a control group of children from the same State [13]. The usual inference from this study is that the virtual elimination of sugar from the diet drastically reduced the level of dental decay [9]. However, it is usual for children living under communal conditions to have a lower caries rate, since between-meal foods, whether sugar or starch based, are not available [10].

Turku Xylitol Study

A large-scale dietary study was carried out in Turku, Finland, in which xylitol, an artifical sweetener, was used to replace sugar in the diet [14]. The rationale was that the xylitol was a substance not fermented by oral plaque organisms. In the study 125 subjects, aged 15 to 45 years, were divided into three groups: one group used sucrose in their diet, a second replaced sucrose with fructose and in a third group sucrose was replaced by xylitol. After 2 years there was a slightly lower caries rate, based upon cavitation, in the fructose group whereas the xylitol group had a lower level of caries by 56%. It should be noted that many of the subjects were in an age group where caries would be expected to be low, but this research showed that the substitution of sucrose by a substance that oral bacteria cannot ferment, led to significantly lower caries incidence. However, it also showed that there was little difference between sucrose and fructose in cariogenic potential.

Studies in North America

In the United States many studies have been concerned with the possible association between sucrose and dental caries. Recent reports have shown that no significant relationship exists for breakfast cereals [15] or for sugar and confectionery [16,91,92], but that there is a significant relationship between caries and frequency of sucrose consumption [93]. In a recent paper Ismail [17] reported on Americans aged 9 to 29 years examined for the first National Health and Nutrition Survey. Individuals with a DMFT score equal to or above the 80th percentile were compared with those below the 20th percentile. The strongest discriminator between high and low decay was between-meal consumption of table sugars and syrups. The use of breakfast cereals, bread and fruit juices, icecream, nuts and biscuits was not associated with a high decay rate, perhaps because they were found to be consumed only infrequently.

Studies in the United Kingdom

A similar study to that of Ismail's was carried out in the United Kingdom by Rugg-Gunn [18] using a prospective dietary record for some 400 children in Northumberland over several years. Dental caries incidence was monitored and related to the quantity, frequency and type of sugars consumed. Results showed that sugar consumption and frequency were not significantly related to dental caries except in those children with the highest increment of decay. These children had a significantly higher consumption of between-meal, sugary snacks, and total sugar consumption was more strongly correlated with caries incidence than was frequency for the high caries subjects. No such relationship was found for the bulk of the study population. The statistical correlations reported were not strong and the reported frequency of sugar intake was low. The overall association was therefore weak. The implications were that sucrose restriction be advocated largely for those individuals who had a high risk of dental caries.

South African Studies

Studies in South Africa concerning the relationship of caries to sugar consumption have been very controversial. In pre-school children in South Africa, Cleaton-Jones et al. [19] found an association between dental caries prevalence and the consumption of sugary foods. However Sundin et al. [20] questioned whether any such relationship could be validly shown. Ismail [17] felt that such studies based upon 24-hour recall of a diet seriously underestimated the usual consumption of carbohydrate by about one third, as deduced from the studies of Beaton et al. [21]. Other reports on the different racial groups in South Africa have led to the conclusion that genetic and immunological factors may be of greater importance than sugar ingestion [19,22,23]. These findings have not been generally accepted.

   More recently, also in South Africa, Steyn et al. [24] completed a dietary and dental survey of 12-year-old white, coloured, black and Indian children. Dietary data were again based upon a 24-hour recall. Overall correlations between total sucrose intake and dental decay were not significant. The decay rate, expressed as DMFT, was correlated with frequency of sucrose intake.

Frequency of Consumption

The frequency of eating sucrose, and other carbohydrates, is directly proportional to the incidence of dental caries [25,26]. Animal experiments, discussed more fully below, support this relationship [20,30]. Burt [31] felt that frequency might be important in communities where sugar consumption was low, but less so in industrialised countries where there was a generally high intake. However, for the at-risk individual there certainly seems to be a significant relationship between caries and frequency of eating sucrose.

Reliability of Diet Studies

All of the above human studies have depended on recall of food consumption. Obviously such studies rely on the accuracy of recall by the subjects [21], or what they report as eaten. In addition, if foods under study are usually consumed with an extra amount of table sugar, syrup or other natural sweetener, then failure to account for the consumption of the added sugars may lead to errors in the analysis. In the study by Ismail [17] the consumption of coffee, chocolate and tea drinks was associated, in a regression model, with high levels of dental decay. When an account was made of the same-day consumption of added table sugars the association disappeared.

Evidence from Animal Studies

Because human studies have been difficult, and intervention studies ethically questionable, many researchers have turned towards the use of experimental animals to test for the cariogenicity of foods. The animal model has many advantages. The laboratory rat is used for most experiments, which enables a pure-bred strain of animal to be tested. Meals can be programmed so that the size of meals consumed, the intervals between meals and the frequency of eating can all be controlled [27]. The experimental design allows for a standard oral organism, usually *Streptococcus mutans*, to be the same for all animals. Water, temperature and humidity can all be controlled. There have now been well over 30 reports on the cariogenicity of food tested by the animal model. The more recent studies comparing sugars and starches in foods are of particular interest. Grenby and Paterson [32] showed there were twice as many carious lesions in rats fed cooked biscuit than in a group fed uncooked sugar and flour. When sugar was baked into biscuits the caries incidence rose significantly. Further experiments by Grenby and Bull [33], using baked biscuits versus unbaked biscuits or biscuits without sugar, confirmed these findings. Other animal studies have confirmed the high cariogenicity of sucrose [34,35]. Pre-sweetened breakfast cereals have also been shown to produce higher caries in the rat [36].

Bowen et al. [37] reported that starch had about 45% of the cariogenicity of sucrose, and that breakfast cereals containing 8%, 14% or 60% sucrose were of nearly equal cariogenicity. The test method of Bowen used 17 snacks fed to rats in a programmed feeding machine. To avoid the possibility of the essential nutrients having an effect on the prevalence of dental caries, the diet was given by gastric lavage, and therefore only the test snack foods touched the teeth. This method was accepted as a valid one for the testing of the cariogenic potential of foods [41]. Using a similar experimental design Mundorff et al. [38] showed that a number of foods, containing various types of starches, had a cariogenic potential. Mundorff and Curzon [39] found that starchy foods could have as much as 87% of the cariogenicity of sucrose. Potato crisps were highly variable in their effect, scoring as low as 40% but as high as 93% of the cariogenicity of sucrose. A frequency–sucrose–starch interrelationship therefore affects dental caries as demonstrated in the many animal experiments.

Some researchers dismiss animal experiments as unreliable [40]. Firstly, animals may not like the foods tested. Secondly, in the rat, the saliva composition is quite different from that of man, being high in phosphate. This would materially affect the rate of caries formation. Thirdly, in order to standardise experimental conditions, rats are super-infected with cariogenic organisms, and this artificial condition may affect a food comparison. Finally, virtually all experiments that have been reported have tested single foods against each other, whereas in man meals or snacks always consist of mixtures of foods. On the other hand the animal model using the rat is simple, so that many research laboratories throughout the world are able to undertake such experiments. The methodology is cheap and very rapidly produces reliable results within a few weeks. Many scientists accept the limitations of the methods but

Table 4.1.   Snack foods with low cariogenic potential

Nuts	Peanuts, brazils, cashews, mixed nuts
Crisps, corn and potato snacks	Plain and flavoured (e.g. cheese and onion, Bovril, bacon, Hula Hoops, Horror Bags, Ringos: check the ingredients list for sugar, but most brands do not have sugar)
Savoury biscuits	Ryvita, water biscuits, Cheeselets, Tuc, crispbreads
Savoury spreads	Any cheese or cheese spreads, cold meats, meat and fish pastes, Marmite, liver sausage
Bread	Brown, wholemeal or white – sliced or as rolls; with added fibre is best
Cereals	Porridge oats, Shredded Wheat, Puffed Wheat, wheatgerm, Grapenuts (if it is a snack, do not put sugar on!)
Fruit	Oranges, bananas, pears, plums, tangerines, apples, apricots, pineapple, pomegranates (but avoid very frequent intake)
Vegetables	Carrots, cucumber, tomatoes, cabbage, celery and other vegetables – can be prepared attractively
Other snacks	Plain and low calorie/low fat yoghurt, sugarless gum, sugar-free sweets
Drinks	Tea, milk, coffee (without added sugar) Diet Pepsi, sugarfree squash, Bitter Lemon, 1-Cal Coke, unsweetened fruit juices (avoid frequent intake)

consider that while unable to extrapolate values for relative cariogenicity causally, they can ascribe similarly ranked food cariogenicity for humans [41]. Nevertheless the cariogenic potential of a food as determined by the animal method is indicative of its likely effect on caries in man [42]. Tables of snack foods of low cariogenic potential have therefore been produced (Table 4.1) for recommending to at-risk subjects.

Plaque pH Experiments

When oral bacteria ferment dietary carbohydrate, acids (lactic, acetic and others) are produced. If the pH in the plaque then drops below 5.5, enamel apatite starts to dissolve. Measurement of plaque pH below this "critical pH" has therefore been a method of assessing the cariogenic potential of foods since Stephan [43] first undertook such experiments. The method, which was initially rather crudely carried out with hand-held electrodes, has now been developed to a high degree of reliability [44] and is widely used [45]. With the addition of radio telemetry [46] it shows great promise. Criticism of the research has repeatedly noted that the method measures only the acid present and is not an assessment of dental caries. Nevertheless many scientists are prepared to accept it for the evaluation of foods [42].

Plaque pH experiments have shown sucrose to produce low pH readings, well below the critical pH of 5.5, but so also have a number of starches [47,48]. On the evidence of these researchers it has been claimed that starches in the diet must be considered cariogenic, though not to the same degree as sucrose [47]. Therefore the form of a dietary carbohydrate affects its cariogenicity.

Carbohydrate Type and its Effect on Cariogenicity

Carbohydrate occurs in a number of different forms: as sugars, such as sucrose, fructose and maltose, or as starches, such as wheat, maize, rice, potato or sago. Cooking of raw starch causes the plant cells to swell and break up, releasing starch which can then be further degraded to give monosaccharides. Such degradation can occur in the mouth in the initial stages when starch is broken down to maltose, although this is only transitory.

In any discussion of dental caries the major form of carbohydrate for consideration is sugar as sucrose. There is no dispute that sucrose is a major cause of dental caries when used frequently. While some authors maintain that only sucrose is the "arch enemy" [2,49,50], others do not accept this [51], or they feel that other forms of carbohydrate may also be responsible for dental caries [31,41,52,53].

The issues that merit further discussion are whether sucrose is the sole cause of caries, whether the total quantity of sucrose used is relevant, whether the frequency of use is more important than total consumption, and whether there is a crucial threshold level of sucrose usage. Quantity and frequency have already been referred to, but the question of a critical threshold level remains to be considered.

Threshold Levels of Sugars

Related to the findings of the various epidemiologic studies in man, attempts have been made to devise a threshold level for sugar consumption. Newbrun [55,56], Sheiham [49] and Sreebny [11] have all suggested threshold levels. Recommendations have been made that 50 grams per person per day should be the accepted limit [11], or more broadly that sucrose use should be reduced by half [57].

Most Western societies have average consumption levels many times in excess of the suggested threshold level, and there is no evidence that a reduction in sugar consumption to the suggested thresholds would lead to any appreciable reduction in caries [3]. In those industrialised countries where there has been a substantial reduction in caries during the past decade, overall intake of fermentable carbohydrate has remained static [59]. In the United States, per capita use of sugars has remained steady from 1920 to 1971 [58]. Although dietary habits may have changed, there has not been a dramatic fall in the amount of sugary foods eaten. Nor is there evidence that the pattern of consumption has been radically modified in a favourable way [60]. Indeed in the United States there is evidence that the frequency of eating has gone up [61]. This decline in caries has been related to the extensive use of preventive measures, such as fluoride [62], rather than to any changes in dietary habits. Animal experiments have shown that not only is the frequency of eating sucrose more important than the quantity but also that the interval between snacks is relevant [28]. It is only when the quantity/frequency rate drops to well below half that any substantial reduction in dental caries occurs. This confirms the many findings from human studies that caries activity may be related more to the number of times that between-meal eating occurs [63].

A threshold level of sucrose consumption is therefore not supported by any scientific evidence. While it may be important for an individual who is caries-prone to avoid a large total intake and frequency of sucrose consumption, there is no need for arbitrary guidelines for the whole population.

Natural Versus Refined Carbohydrates

The natural sugars, sucrose, fructose, lactose and glucose, are all cariogenic. Indeed experimental evidence from an analysis of many snack foods found that the statistically significant correlation of caries prevalence was to glucose concentration [39]. The Turku xylitol study showed that when cavitation was used as a measure of dental decay, there was virtually no difference in cariogenicity between sucrose and fructose [10].

The unrefined diet of primitive man was of low cariogenicity [64]. Cereals, fruits and vegetables have all been shown to be cariogenic, but the current argument concerns the degree of cariogenicity. It has been claimed that sugar cane, when chewed, has low cariogenic potential because of its high fibre content [65,66], but this is not always so [67].

Honey is highly cariogenic as it contains mostly fructose and glucose [68]. Other sources of natural sugars are fresh fruits, dried fruits, fruit juices and drinks, all of which have a varying degree of cariogenicity. Fructose, from fruit, is as cariogenic as sucrose. The manner of using fruit, the retentiveness in the mouth, and water content, are such as to make fresh fruit, as normally used, of relatively low cariogenic potential. However, in a number of recent studies dried fruits, particularly raisins, have been shown to be highly cariogenic [37,39,78], although Rugg-Gunn, in an extensive review, disputes this [40]. Nevertheless dried fruits have been implicated in so many experiments on dental caries that one must seriously question advocating them as safe snacks for children.

Lactose, or milk sugar, can be used by oral bacteria for energy production. In infants a type of caries involving the primary incisors has been described by a number of authors [69,70]. In these case reports prolonged, on-demand breast feeding gave rise to a rapid destruction of the primary teeth. Experimental evidence has shown that milk, either human or bovine, can bring about enamel dissolution [71]. Lactose is therefore fermentable by dental plaque and must be considered cariogenic. Obviously the opportunity for lactose to be cariogenic is limited and this sugar should not be considered as a major factor in the causation of caries. Nevertheless it illustrates the point that all types of sugars have a cariogenic potential.

Starch

Cereal products are now thought to play a role in the causation of dental caries [41]. Throughout history, even as far back as the Third Dynasty in Egypt, caries incidence has been found in populations who have used sieved wheat flour in their diets, and there is an association of starches with caries wherever wheat is the main cereal used [72].

There is obviously a distinction to be made between raw and cooked starches. In vitro studies have clearly shown that plaque pH in the human mouth is not depressed when raw wheat, or other raw starches, are eaten [72], but cereals are seldom eaten raw and are usually cooked. Even when no sugar has been added, which is rare in Western cultures, cooking practices produce temperatures which gelatinise starch in the starch-rich foods. Such a change enables the starch to be used by oral bacteria. In the industrial process many cereals are changed, so altering their cariogenic potential.

In a recent study in South Africa [73] the cariogenicity of cooked and uncooked home-prepared maize, factory-milled maize and factory-milled sorghum was evaluated against control groups of rats fed cooked wheat starch and sucrose and maize plus sucrose. The maize and sorghum, whether cooked or uncooked, had a low cariogenicity, but the addition of only 20% sucrose increased the caries prevalence. Others have also shown this [34], and in vivo plaque pH studies have also indicated a cariogenic potential for starches [47].

In many parts of the world wheat is not the staple starch used. Studies by Schamschula et al. [74] in Papua New Guinea showed high caries rates in the Sepik River people consuming diets high in cooked sago. By contrast rice, whether cooked or uncooked, appears to be of low cariogenicity [40]. Rice, potatoes and pasta clear more rapidly from the mouth than other cooked starches, such as bread. The clearance time of starches may affect whether or not they have any cariogenic potential [75], and the presence of starch could also increase the retentiveness of sucrose in the mouth. Substantial drops in plaque pH occur after chewing bread, and/or having a 1% rinse of wheat starch [47].

Other Factors Affecting the Cariogenicity of Carbohydrate

Food characteristics affecting the cariogenicity of a food include chemical composition, caries-inhibiting factors, and physical and organoleptic considerations. These include particle size, solubility, detergent components, and texture. The length of time that a carbohydrate is present in the mouth will therefore determine its cariogenicity.

Any food will stick to the teeth to a greater or lesser degree. The Vipeholm study showed that the more retentive a food the greater was its cariogenic potential [12]. Retentiveness is based upon a food's composition, texture, solubility and effect on saliva flow. Bibby et al. [76] showed that the addition of fat to a food markedly changed its retentiveness. Thus butter increased the rate at which bread was cleared from the mouth. Morrissey et al [77] showed that raisins were highly retentive and that this accounted for their cariogenicity. Foods with a low retention, and often a high fat content, such as cheese, have a low cariogenicity [48].

However, foods may contain caries inhibitors. Fluoride is an obvious example, and the concentration of this element is significantly related to the cariogenic potential of a food [39]. Phosphates [79], trace elements [80] and fatty acids [81] are all cariostatic agents. Other food components such as vanillin, tannins, xanthines, caffeine and theobromines may have anticariogenic abilities, and it has been suggested that one reason for the relatively low cariogenic potential of chocolate is due to components of the cocoa bean [82]. Similarly liquorice has a low caries-promoting ability, ascribed to glycyrrhizinic acid [83]. Part of this inhibition may be of plaque formation, or it may bring about changes in the physical properties of a food and hence its clearance time from the mouth.

Starch products have clearance times as long as 20–30 minutes (for bread and crackers) [84] which may be affected by the gluten content [3]. Changing the contact time of a sucrose-containing food may alter its cariogenicity. Methods of increasing the clearance time of food are used for dental health education. By advocating brushing of the teeth after eating, use of detergent foods (raw vegetables), or eating cheese and nuts at the end of a meal, retention of cariogenic foods in the mouth is reduced.

Assessment of the Cariogenic Potential of Foods

As dental caries is the result of an interaction between dietary carbohydrate, cariogenic oral flora and the tooth substance (host), so the environmental challenge (bacteria–substrate reaction) is an important variable in the process. Even those teeth which have been well formed within an optimal fluoride environment, and with a continuous supply of topical fluoride, may still succumb to the challenge of a diet high in fermentable carbohydrate. With the drop in the prevalence of dental caries in many countries, there remain individuals who are still caries-prone [42]. It is to these at-risk individuals that counselling on cariogenic dietary carbohydrate is directed.

Reliable methods for estimating the potential cariogenicity of foods are needed to assist in providing sound dietary advice. While there have been many attempts to devise a method for determining the cariogenic potential of foods [85], no single method has been widely accepted [42]. The plaque pH method of Graf and Muhlemann [44], used in Switzerland, has been developed to a high degree of sophistication by Schachtele and Jensen [48]. This method is by no means widely accepted.

The animal model using the rat in the programmed feeding machine [27] has been suggested as the only reliable method for testing cariogenicity [37]. While this strong statement has much evidence to support it, other researchers have voiced the opinion that any results of animal experiments cannot be directly extrapolated to man [40]. This view is now confined to only a small group of scientists who are wedded to the validity of the human dietary survey; most researchers accept the animal model as indicative of the likely effects of a food on caries in man [86].

Following the International Consensus Conference on the Cariogenicity of Foods in 1985 [87], an agreement was achieved to accept a combination of the three methods for testing cariogenicity of foods: (1) plaque pH profile (in human experiments); (2) ability to dissolve enamel (in vitro); (3) production of caries in animals. The results derived from the three methods provide an acceptable Cariogenic Potential Index (CPI) for any particular food.

Results from experiments using these methods [33,37,38,44,47,48,78] show that most foods containing dietary carbohydrate can be cariogenic. Fruit sugars, sucrose, starches and combinations thereof are all more or less cariogenic. Relatively few foods are of negligible effect on caries.

While a three-method integrated selection procedure might indicate a carbohydrate was highly cariogenic, is this enough for our needs? It might be acceptable for dental clinicians and dental researchers to say food A was "highly cariogenic" or food B was "safe for teeth", but how should we categorise other foods? Would the majority fall into the middle ground?

As shown in Fig. 4.1 a series of tests of CPI, using the animal model, differentiated between very high and very low cariogenic foods, but could not discriminate between a large group of snack foods in the middle range [38]. Similarly the plaque pH telemetry studies of Schachtele and Jensen [48] showed that most foods, as eaten, depressed plaque pH while only the foods of extremely low CPI – aged cheddar cheese and skimmed milk – did not.

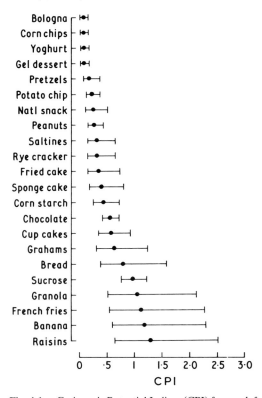

Fig. 4.1. Cariogenic Potential Indices (CPI) for snack foods based on smooth surface caries in rats compared with sucrose. (After Mundorff et al. [38].)

A further reason for a lack of discrimination is the variability of the CPI of carbohydrate foods even under similar test conditions. Some apparently paradoxical results have been noted for similar foods when tested by different workers [3]. Recently, however, it has been shown that CPI scores may vary for a food even under identical test conditions [39]. This has been suggested to be due to variables in the maufacture of the foods which may be seasonal or economic. Grenby [88] has shown that the degree of processing of foods affects their cariogenicity and may vary from season to season, and from month to month. The more a carbohydrate is processed, or perhaps the more refined the carbohydrate, the greater its cariogenicity. When similar foods were tested by two of the three methods outlined above, results for individual test foods were close, but discrimination was poor [87].

Evaluation of the Cariogenicity of Dietary Carbohydrates

Plaque pH Measurements

Most foods containing fermentable carbohydrate cause a marked decrease in the pH of interproximal plaque (the plaque lodged between the teeth) [89], but the minimum

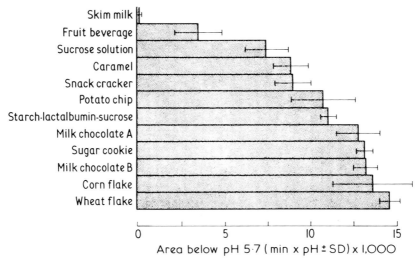

Fig. 4.2. Effects of various foods on plaque pH depression measured by indwelling electrode. (After Schactele and Jensen [48].)

pH is reached after varying periods of time [48]. Plotting pH response against time, the area of the graph below pH 5.7 (critical pH) can be calculated and used to rank foods according to the *duration* of the period when the hydrogen ion concentration is sufficiently low to cause acid dissolution of the enamel [90]. Using this approach Schachtele and Jensen [48] ranked their 13 test foods into five groups ranging from the least to the most acidogenic:

Group 1: aged Cheddar cheese
Group 2: skimmed milk
Group 3: 10% sucrose solution and fruit beverage
Group 4: caramel, cracker, potato crisps, starch–lactalbumin–sucrose (SLS)
Group 5: milk chocolate, sugar cookie (biscuit), corn flakes and wheat flakes

A close look at the results, as reproduced in Fig. 4.2, shows that if the overlap of the standard deviations is used as a means of differentiating significantly between foods, then the groups become:

1. Aged Cheddar cheese and non-fat dry milk solution
2. Fruit beverage
3. Sucrose solution, caramel, snack cracker, potato crisps, SLS
4. Milk chocolate (A and B), sugar cookie (biscuit), corn flakes and wheat flakes

This discrimination into four groups can be compared with the rat caries study of Mundorff et al. [38], where only three groups of foods could be identified by CPI (Fig. 4.1.; see above). It is of note, however, that in these pH studies all foods containing dietary carbohydrate produced a plaque pH below the critical 5.5. Only foods such as cheese high in fat and skimmed milk did not lead to an acidogenic response. It must be emphasised that these pH tests do not produce dental caries, and therefore the results cannot be used as showing a causal relationship between dietary carbohydrate and caries.

Animal Caries

The rat caries model attempts to produce dental caries using experimental conditions where microflora, enamel, substrate and time are all present. The disadvantage of this method is that the test does not use a human mouth and results cannot be *directly extrapolated* to man. However, if the experiment is properly designed results can be *applied to man* [86]. As with the pH electrode studies, substantial numbers of carbohydrate foods have now been tested. Extensive lists of CPI scores are available [28,38,78,86]. Just as a study of the plaque pH results (Fig. 4.2) showed considerable overlap of standard deviations, there are similar problems with results from rat caries studies as shown in Fig. 4.1. If these findings are considered critically then only those foods containing dietary carbohydrate at the two extremes of the scales can be separated. The study of Mundorff et al. [38] showed three groups of foods:

1. Bologna (meat sausage), corn chips (crisps), yoghurt, jello dessert (jelly)
2. Pretzels, potato chips (crisps), Natural Snac (nuts and dried fruit), peanuts, saltines (cream crackers), rye crackers, fried cake, sponge cake, corn starch, chocolate, bread
3. Raisins, bananas, french fries, granola (oat crunch)

Foods based on corn (maize) starches, and high in fluoride, have a low degree of cariogenicity while foods such as cakes and dried fruits which are high in glucose and sucrose are of high cariogenicity.

Consumption Patterns

Are there interactions between cariogenicity and frequency of consumption, quantity consumed and time of day that need to be tested? Frequency is a major factor in determining the cariogenicity of a food and this parameter is taken into account in the animal caries model with programmed feeding, as is the quantity of food used [37]. This is not usually evaluated in the majority of plaque pH experiments. In due course the indwelling electrode plaque pH method will need to be used to assess foods in the light of food combinations and consumption patterns, perhaps when radio telemetry has been perfected [46].

Acceptance of Methods

Worldwide there have been varying degrees of acceptance of the necessary methodology for assessing the cariogenicity of dietary carbohydrate. There has been the official use of a single method, interdental plaque pH by indwelling electrode, as in Switzerland. However, no other country has followed this example with a CPI method recognised by a government body. In other countries, such as Great Britain, acceptance of the need for a method will depend on a decision not by government but by some body such as the UK Health Education Authority, which was campaigning actively for an improvement in diet but has no plans to approve official testing of the cariogenicity of dietary carbohydrates. It may well be that an approach by a government agency would be unacceptable to many scientists, yet the development of a consensus by dental researchers, in collaboration with the food industry, would probably achieve a much wider acceptance than directives of a government body based on a limited, and self-perpetuating, group of dental authorities.

Dietary Carbohydrate in a Balanced Diet

Unfortunately there is still disagreement and discord between dental scientists as to the role of dietary carbohydrates on dental caries. Some dental researchers consider that only sucrose needs controlling, if not eliminating, in the diet. A balanced diet would therefore not include sucrose in any form. Others believe that all dietary carbohydrates should be thought of as cariogenic, and that it is the form and method of use that should be stressed in advising people who wish to reduce their susceptibility to dental decay. Frequency of exposure to dietary carbohydrates is just as important as the quantity used. While not advocating the dictatorial use of foods "friendly to teeth", which might promote a philosophy of dietary celibacy, we must be aware that such recommendations would not be applicable or acceptable to all individuals. With a list of recommended foods the individual would have choices based upon sound scientific assessment.

In recent years the weight of opinion in the dental scientific community has evolved to the point of view that most dietary carbohydrates are potentially cariogenic. Many dietary carbohydrates pose a risk to the individual who is caries-prone. Frequent use of fruits and starches will increase the risk of decay. Correspondingly, however, there are many people with a high resistance to decay who may freely use most dietary carbohydrates without risk.

In categorising dietary carbohydrate, therefore, we must consider three groups of foods. Those in the first group are of such negligible cariogenic potential as to pose no risk to anybody. Examples are cheese, nuts and some foods based on maize. A second, very large group, contains foods of low risk to the bulk of the population, but which may pose a danger to people of high caries susceptibility. Finally, the third group includes those foods that are highly cariogenic to most of the population. This group includes sucrose sweets, dried fruits, starch–sucrose combinations which are very retentive, and acid foods.

Summary

Dietary carbohydrates are an essential part of the balanced diet. The type, composition and frequency of use of foods must all be taken into account when counselling patients with dental caries on the use of carbohydrates, as both sugars and starches having a degree of cariogenicity. All the common sugars are cariogenic, but under certain conditions sucrose is more so than others. Only because sucrose is the sugar eaten most often can it be regarded as uniquely associated with caries. In preventing dental caries the most effective method remains the use of fluoridated water as well as the use of fluoride toothpaste. The ability to bring about major changes in the diet of both individuals and populations is very limited and would not be cost-effective. In advanced industrialised countries such as the United Kingdom, a reduction of dietary carbohydrate, as sucrose, in the diet is probably unattainable, and unnecessary with the use of fluoride.

References

1. Bejam Ltd (1985) Market report on housewives' attitudes to frozen food use and food labelling. Bejam Ltd, London
2. Newbrun E (1969) Sucrose, the arch criminal of dental caries. J Dent Child 36:239–248
3. Bibby BG (1975) The cariogenicity of snack foods and confections. J Am Dent Assoc 90:121–132
4. Bibby BG (1983) Changing perspectives on dental caries. In: Story E (ed) Diet and dental caries; changing perspectives. University of Melbourne Press, Melbourne
5. Curzon MEJ, Curzon JA (1970) Dental caries in Eskimo children of the Keewatin District of the Northwest Territories. J Can Dent Assoc 36:342–345
6. Tovrud G (1957) Influence of war and post-war conditions on the teeth of Norwegian schoolchildren. III. Discussion of food supply and dental conditions in Norway and other European countries. Milbank Q 35:373–382
7. Takeuchi M (1961) Epidemiological study on dental caries in Japanese children – before, during and after World War II. Int Dent J 11:443–445
8. Marthaler T (1967) Epidemiological and clinical dental findings in relation to intake of carbohydrates. Caries Res 1:222–228
9. Murray JJ (ed) (1983) The prevention of dental disease. Oxford University Press, Oxford
10. Nikiforuk G (1985) Understanding dental caries. I. Etiology and mechanisms: basic aspects. Karger, Basel
11. Sreebny LM (1982) Sugar availability, sugar consumption and dental caries. Community Dent Oral Epidemiol 10:1–7
12. Gustafson BE et al. (1954) The Vipeholm dental caries study. The effect of different levels of carbohydrate intake on caries activity in 436 individuals observed for five years. Acta Odontol Scand 11:232–240
13. Sullivan HR, Harris RM (1958) The biology of the children in Hopewood House, Bowral, New South Wales. II. Observations extending over five years (1952–1956). 2. Observations on oral conditions. Aust Dent J 3:311–317
14. Scheinin A, Makinen KK (1975) Turku sugar studies I–XXI. Acta Odontol Scand 70:1–350
15. Glass RL, Fleisch S (1974) Diet and caries: dental caries incidence and the consumption of ready to eat cereals. J Am Dent Assoc 88:807–813
16. Bagramian RA et al. (1974) Diet patterns and dental caries in third grade US children. Community Dent Oral Epidemiol 2:208–213
17. Ismail AI (1986) Food cariogenicity in Americans aged from 9 to 29 years in a national cross-sectional survey, 1971–1974. J Dent Res 65:1435–1440
18. Rugg-Gunn AJ et al. (1984) Relationship between dietary habits and caries increment assessed over two years in 405 English adolescent school children. Arch Oral Biol 29:983–992
19. Cleaton-Jones P et al. (1984) Dental caries and sucrose intake in five South African preschool groups. Community Dent Oral Epidemiol 12:381–385
20. Sundin B, Birkhead D, Granath L (1983) Is there not a strong relationship nowadays between caries and consumption of sweets? Swed Dent J 7:103–108
21. Beaton GH et al. (1979) Sources of variance in the 24-hour dietary recall data: implications for nutrition study design and interpretation. Am J Clin Nutr 32:2546–2559
22. Richardson BD et al. (1978) Total sucrose intake and dental caries in Black and in White South African children of 1–6 years. I. Sucrose intake. J Dent Assoc S Africa 33:533–537
23. Walker APR (1984) How predictable are meaningful reductions in dental caries by dietary means? Nutr Abstr Rev 54:211–217
24. Steyn NP et al. (1987) Sucrose consumption and dental caries in twelve-year-old children of all ethnic groups residing in Cape Town. J Dent Assoc S Africa 42:43–49
25. Clancy KL et al. (1977) Snack food intake of adolescents and caries development. J Dent Res 56:568–573
26. Burt BA et al. (1982) Diet and dental health, a study of relationships: United States, 1971–1974. National Centre for Health Statistics: series 11, no. 225. US Government Printing Office, Washington
27. Konig KG, Schmid P, Schmid R (1968) An apparatus for frequency controlled feeding of small rodents and its use in dental caries experiments. Arch Oral Biol 13:13–26
28. Bowen WH et al. (1983) Effect of varying intervals between meals on dental caries in rats. Caries Res 17:466–471

29. Firestone AR, Imfeld T, Schmid R, Muhlemann HR (1980) Cariogenicity of foods. J Am Dent Assoc 101:443–444
30. Steckson-Blicks C, Arvidsson S, Holm A-K (1985) Dental health, dental care and dietary habits in children in different parts of Sweden. Acta Odontol Scand 43:59–67
31. Burt BA (1985) The future of the caries decline. J. Public Health Dent 45:261–269
32. Grenby TH, Paterson FM (1972) Effect of sweet biscuits on the incidence of dental caries in rats. Br J Nutr 27:195–199
33. Grenby TH, Bull JM (1977) Three ways of making sweet biscuits less harmful to the teeth. In: Birch GG, Shallenberger RS (eds) Developments in food carbohydrate, vol 1. Applied Science Publishers, London
34. Hefti A, Schmid R (1979) Effect on caries incidence in rats of increasing dietary sucrose levels. Caries Res. 13:298–300
35. Michalek SM et al. (1977) Low sucrose levels promote extensive *Streptococcus mutans*-induced dental caries. Infect Immun 16:712–714
36. McDonald JL, Stookey GK (1977) Animal studies concerning the cariogenicity of dry breakfast cereals. J Dent Res 56:1001–1006
37. Bowen WH et al. (1980) A method of assessing cariogenic potential of foodstuffs. J Am Dent Assoc 100:677–681
38. Mundorff SA et al. (1985) Cariogenicity of foods: rat study. IADR Abstract 64: No. 1071, Las Vegas, USA
39. Mundorff SA, Curzon MEJ (1985) Variation in the cariogenicity of snack foods when tested under identical experimental conditions. J Paediatr Dent 1:71–75
40. Rugg-Gunn AJ (1986) Starchy foods and fresh fruits: their relative importance as a source of dental caries in Britain. Health Educational Council, London (Occasional Paper No. 3)
41. Tanzer JM (1985) Testing food cariogenicity with experimental animals. In: Scientific consensus conference on methods for the assessment of the cariogenic potential of foods. San Antonio, Texas, 1985
42. Curzon MEJ (1986) Integration of methods for determining the cariogenic potential of foods: is this possible with present technology? J Dent Res 65:1520–1524
43. Stephan RM (1940) Changes in hydrogen ion concentration on tooth surfaces and in carious lesions. J Am Dent Assoc 27:718–723
44. Graf H, Muhlemann HR (1966) Telemetry of plaque pH from interdental areas. Helv Odontol Acta 10:94–101
45. Geddes DAM (1984) Current view of plaque acidogenicity. In: Cariology today. Proceedings of the International Congress, Zurich, 1983. Karger, Basle
46. Armstrong WG, Wells PJ (1987) Continuous in vivo telemetric measurement of human interproximal plaque acid production caused by dietary components. 34th ORCA Congress, Budapest, 1987 (Abstract No. 72)
47. Morman JE, Muhlemann HR (1981) Oral starch degradation and its influence on acid production in human dental plaque. Caries Res 15:166–175
48. Schachtele CF, Jensen ME (1984) Can foods be ranked according to their cariogenic potential? In: Cariology today. Proceedings of the international congress, Zurich, 1983. Karger, Basel, pp 136–146
49. Sheiham A (1983) Sugars and dental decay. Lancet I:282–284
50. Rugg-Gunn AJ, Edgar WM (1984) Sugar and dental caries – a review of the evidence. Community Dent Health 1:85–92
51. Walker ARP (1986) Diet and dental caries: a sceptical view. Am J Clin Nutr 43:969–971
52. Navia JM (1977) Animal models in dental research. University of Alabama Press, Birmingham, Alabama
53. Alfano MC (1982) Changing concepts of diet and dental caries. In: Story E (ed) Diet and dental caries. Proceedings of symposium, Melbourne, 1982
54. Hardwick JL (1960) The incidence and distribution of caries throughout the ages in relation to the Englishman's diet. Br Dent J 108:9–17
55. Newbrun E (1979) Dietary carbohydrates: their role in cariogenicity. Med Clin North Am 63:1069–1086
56. Newbrun E (1982) Sugar and dental caries: a review of human studies. Science 217:418–423
57. British Nutrition Foundation (1986) Sugars and syrups task force: conclusions and recommendations. British Nutrition Foundation, London
58. Page L, Friend B (1974) Level of use of sugars in the United States. In: Sipple H, McNutt KW (eds) Sugars in nutrition. Academic Press, New York
59. Groeneveld A et al. (1987) Caries experience of 15-year-old children in Tiel and Culemborg after cessation of water fluoridation. 34th annual ORCA conference, 1987 (Abstract No. 63)
60. Naylor MN (1985) Possible factors underlying the decline in caries prevalence. J R Soc Med 78:23–25

61. Holm A-K, Theilade E, Birkhead D (1986) Dietary measures and dental caries. In: Thylstrup A, Fejerskov O (eds) Textbook of cariology. Munksgaard, Copenhagen
62. Ainamo J (1987) The decline of dental caries in European countries. In: Frank RM, O'Hickey S (eds) Strategy for dental caries prevention in European countries. Proceedings of an international symposium. IRL Press, Oxford, pp 21–36
63. Weis RL, Trihart AH (1960) Between meal eating habits and dental caries experience in pre-school children. Am J Public Health 61:1097–1099
64. Jenkins GN (1981) Nutrition and caries. Proc Finn Dent Soc 77:183–187
65. Kunzel W et al. (1973) Auswirkungen habituellen Zuckerrohrkauens auf Kariesbefall und Parodontalzustand Kubenischer Zuckerrohrarbeiter. Dtsch Stomatol 23:554–561
66. Harris S, Cleaton-Jones P (1978) Oral health of a group of sugarcane chewers. J Dent Assoc S Africa 33:255–258
67. Driezen S, Spies TD (1952) The incidence of dental caries in habitual sugar cane chewers. J Am Dent Assoc 45:193–200
68. Shannon IL, Edmonds EJ, Madsen KO (1979) Honey: sugar content and cariogenicity. J Dent Child 46:29–33
69. Roberts GJ (1982) Is breast feeding a possible cause of dental caries? J Dent 10:346–352
70. Curzon MEJ, Drummond BK (1987) Case report – rampant caries in an infant related to prolonged on-demand breast feeding and a lactovegetarian diet. J Paediatr Dent 3:25–28
71. Rugg-Gunn AJ, Roberts GJ, Wright WG (1985) Effect of human milk on plaque pH in situ and enamel dissolution in vitro compared with bovine milk, lactose and sucrose. Caries Res 19:327–334
72. Bibby BG (1985) Cereal foods and dental caries. Cereal Foods World 30:851–855
73. Schmid R, Cleaton-Jones P, Lutz F (1987) Cariogenicity of uncooked and cooked traditional african foodstuffs in rats. Caries Res 21:339–345
74. Schamschula RG et al. (1978) WHO study of dental caries etiology in Papua New Guinea. WHO, Geneva
75. Krasse B (1985) Caries risk. Quintessence Books, Chicago
76. Bibby BG et al. (1986) Oral food clearance and the pH of plaque and saliva. J Am Dent Assoc 112:333–337
77. Morrissey RB, Burkholder BD, Tarka SM (1984) The cariogenic potential of snack foods. J Am Dent Assoc 109:589–591
78. Navia JM, Lopez H (1983) Rat assay of reference foods and sugar containing snacks. J Dent Res 62:893–898
80. Curzon MEJ (1984) Influence on caries of trace metals other than fluoride. In: Cariology today. Proceedings of the International Congress, Zurich, 1983. Karger, Basle
81. Hayes ML (1981) The inhibition of bacterial glycolysis in human dental plaque by medium-chain fatty acid-sugar mouthwashes. Arch Oral Biol 26:223–227
82. s'Gravenmade EJ, Jenkins GN, Ferguson DB (1977) A potential cariostatic factor in cocoa beans. Caries Res 11:133
83. Edgar M (1978) Reduction in enamel dissolution by liquorice and glycyrrhizinic acid. J Dent Res 57:69–74
84. Lanke LS (1957) Influence on salivary sugar of certain properties of foodstuffs and individual oral conditions. Acta Odontol Scand 15 (Suppl):23
85. Navia JM (1984) The value of animal models to predict the caries-promoting properties of human diet or dietary components. In: Cariology today. Proceedings of the International Congress, Zurich, 1984. Karger, Basel, pp 154–165
86. Tanzer JM (1981) Introduction. In: Tanzer JM (ed) Proceedings of the symposium on animal models in cariology. Special supplement to microbiology abstracts 1981. Information Retrieval Inc, Washington DC (pp 21, Tanzer: Animal models 1981)
87. Harper DS et al. (1985) Dental cariogenic evaluation of foods using human plaque pH and experimental rat caries model. Arch Oral Biol 30:455–460
88. Grenby TH (1985) Dental effects of four different snack foods in laboratory rats. NOF Abstract 64, No. 158. IADR British Division, Warwick
89. Firestone AR et al. (1980) Cariogenicity of foods. J Am Dent Assoc 101:443–444
90. Edgar WM (1982) Methodological considerations affecting the determination of pH in tooth surface plaque. In: Frank RM, Leach SA (eds) Surface and colloid phenomena in the oral cavity. Information Retrieval Inc, Washington DC, pp 131–142
91. Messer LB, Messer HH, Best J (1980) Refined carbohydrate consumption by caries-free and caries-active children. J Dent Res 59 (Special issue B):968 (abstract 324)
92. Bagramian RA, Russell AL (1974) Epidemiologic study of dental caries experience and between meal eating patterns. J Dent Res 52:342–347

93. Hargreaves JA et al. (1980) Dental caries in Canadian children related to between meal sugar consumption. J Dent Res 59 (Special issue B):968 (abstract 325)

Commentary

Southgate: The comment that only caries-prone individuals need to reduce the frequency of sugar consumption is surely only acceptable if some index of caries susceptibility is available that is not dependent on actually having carious lesions.

The use of cariogenicity tests on single foods is only partially informative and clearly can only distinguish the extremes. I personally doubt the value of labelling foods with this property and of the validity of claims for foods being "safe to eat for teeth".

Author's reply: There is limited evidence on the cariogenicity of starch in human populations. The caries in Sepik River New Guinea natives was related to the frequent use of boiled sago. Even so, because starch does not have the same cariogenic potential as sucrose, it is less likely that starch can be shown to be cariogenic in human studies.

Caries-prone individuals can be identified by tests of the buffering capacity and measurement of the *Streptococcus mutans* counts of their saliva. These tests are not entirely reliable, but are now good enough to be used in dental practice.

Rivers: In the Turku xylitol study, did fructose have a significantly lower cariogenic potential than sucrose?

Author's reply: In the Turku study fructose gave a caries rate, as cavitation, only slightly less than that of sucrose. It is generally considered that fructose is cariogenic but not as much as sucrose.

Rivers: In the North American studies it is stated that ice cream and biscuits were consumed "only infrequently" and that that is why no correlation should be expected between frequency of consumption and caries rate. This infrequent consumption does not fit with my prejudices and indeed experiences of American diets. Is the remark correct?

Author's reply: The remark is taken from the paper by Ismail. While one might get the impression that Americans do eat a lot of ice cream, the diet surveys show that this is more often than not with meals and not as between-meal snacks. This is in contrast to other carbohydrate foods. The National Health and Nutrition Survey is considered reliable.

Rivers: Is the metabolic conversion of sucrose and fructose to glucose relevant here? Isn't the relevant point that all these can be fermented in the mouth?

Author's reply: Yes, most sugars (including lactose) can be fermented by oral bacteria in the mouth to give enamel demineralisation

Rivers: What accounted for the variability of the response to potato crisps?

Southgate: The potato tuber is extremely variable and especially so in respect of sugar content. This, coupled with the fact that many potato crisps are reconstituted from potato starch, may be the cause of variable performance in cariogenicity tests. The oil used and the temperature of frying are other possible sources of variability.

MacGregor: What conclusions can be drawn? What would Curzon himself recommend?

Author's reply: The conclusion that can be drawn from a review of dental research on diet and dental caries is that frequency of use of carbohydrate is the major factor determining whether an individual develops dental caries. Subjects who are identified as caries-prone should reduce the frequency of use of foods with a high cariogenic potential.
   Fluoridation of drinking water has been shown to be the most cost-effective method of controlling dental caries. Also effective, but costing more to implement, is the addition of fluoride to toothpaste. Unfortunately, however, only about 55%–60% of the UK population regularly uses fluoride toothpaste. Individual attempts at dietary modification to control dental caries are unlikely to be acceptable or cost-effective.

Macdonald: I thought salivary amylase only broke down carbohydrates to maltose – a disaccharide – and then mostly in the stomach.

Author's reply: Correct, but if starchy foods stay in the mouth for some time, as many foods with slow clearance rates will, then there will be some formation of maltose in the mouth.

Macdonald: Should some mention be made of the claims that milk is anti-cariogenic?

Author's reply: Milk is essentially neutral in its cariogenicity, or rather it does not promote caries unless used excessively frequently, such as with on-demand prolonged breast feeding. However, it is the lactose content of the breast milk that is thought to be cariogenic. When tested in the methods described in the text, milk, usually skimmed milk, does not depress plaque pH and is therefore termed non-cariogenic. This is, however, not quite the same as anti-cariogenic.

Macdonald: I wonder whether it is true that caries is brought about not only by a low pH but by the length of time the pH stays low?

Author's reply: Yes, because a short drop in plaque pH, which rises rapidly back to resting plaque pH, will not bring about much demineralisation of enamel. The saliva in the mouth will rapidly buffer the acid produced and also clear it from the mouth. However, a prolonged depression of pH will lead to a greater amount of demineralisation. It is for this reason that the "area under the curve" in assessing the cariogenicity of a food is considered to be of more importance than the simple drop in pH.

Chapter 5

Salt and Blood Pressure

G. A. MacGregor

Importance of High Blood Pressure

Cardiovascular disease is now the most common cause of death in developed countries. Large-scale population follow-up studies have identified three major risk factors for cardiovascular disease: high blood pressure, high blood lipids and cigarette smoking. Of these three, high blood pressure is now recognised as the most potent predictor of life expectancy, a finding which life insurance companies have recognised for many years. Studies in Western populations have revealed that from 5% to 20% of the population may have high blood pressure, and of those over 95% have essential hypertension, which is to say that the reason for the high blood pressure is not understood. High blood pressure is usually defined, arbitrarily, as a diastolic pressure greater than 90 mmHg and a systolic pressure of greater than 140 mmHg. However, the increased risk of cardiovascular disease is not confined solely to those who have high blood pressure, but is related to the whole range of blood pressure; in other words those people with average blood pressure are at greater risk than those with lower pressures.

There are two major approaches to high blood pressure. One is to try and prevent its development and the other is to wait until it has developed, and then treat it. Much recent evidence now suggests that this second approach does carry benefits, and does reduce the risks, particularly of strokes.

In considering the relationship between salt and blood pressure there are therefore two questions. One is whether a high salt intake in any way causes, precipitates or aggravates the development of high blood pressure, and the second is whether reducing salt intake lowers the raised blood pressure if it has already developed.

Importance of Sodium and Chloride

Sodium and chloride are the two predominant ions in the extracellular space, and thereby play a very important role in regulating the volume of extracellular fluid. The balance, therefore, between sodium and chloride intake and their excretion is critical to the maintenance of extracellular fluid. The amounts of sodium required for normal development are extremely small. Studies of herbivorous mammals living away from the sea, and studies in man, have shown that the body has very powerful mechanisms for conserving sodium and chloride both in the urine and in the sweat [1]. At the same time studies in herbivorous mammals, who obtain all of their sodium and chloride from the very low levels present in the food they eat, have also shown that salt appetite may play an important role in trying to seek out foods with a greater concentration of salt [1]. In man, during evolution and even in some primitive societies today, salt intake only varies between 1 and 20 mmol/day, and some vegetarian communities have intakes of less than 5 mmol/day. This finding is illustrated in very careful studies that have been done in Yanomamö Indians, a tribe living near the Amazon, where 24-hour urinary sodium excretion was only about 1 mmol/day. Studies in this tribe showed that they were in good physical condition, well nourished and very active [1,2].

With increasing civilisation, communities near the sea found that they could evaporate sea water to get salt, and other communities found that salt could be obtained by digging it from the ground. Salt was soon found to act as a preservative, allowing food to be kept during the winter, particularly in northern climates. Salt became of great economic importance, and in many religions was of considerable significance. At the same time many governments used it as a main source of tax revenue. Consumption of salt increased from the comparatively low evolutionary levels of 1–20 mmol/day to the 100–400 mmol/day that is presently consumed. (1 g NaCl = 17 mmol Na^+; 1 g Na^+ = 43.5 mmol Na^+.) It is extremely likely, however, that salt intake was even higher in the late nineteenth century, when it has been estimated that many northern European countries, where salt was widely used as a preservative, may have had sodium intakes varying between 300 and 500 mmol/day, a level roughly equivalent to those a few years ago in the northern islands of Japan. Much circumstantial, and some direct evidence suggests that this still very high consumption of salt may be a predisposing factor to the development of essential hypertension.

Epidemiological Evidence

Studies from less-developed societies where salt is not, or was not, added to the food, have shown that blood pressure does not rise with age, whereas in those societies that do add salt to food, there is a rise in blood pressure with age [3] (Fig. 5.1). Studies where dietary sodium intake has been assessed, or 24-hour urinary sodium excretion measured, have also shown a clear relationship between the prevalence of hypertension in different communities and the amount of sodium consumed or excreted in the urine (Fig. 5.2). However, it must be realised that dietary assessments of sodium intake are not very accurate, that the collection of 24-hour urine samples is difficult, particularly in more primitive communities, and that in Western countries sodium intake varies from day to day [4]. Many of these studies were small or lacked proper controls. Simpson therefore re-analysed what he considered to be the best-controlled of these studies, and again clearly demonstrated that with increasing sodium intake in different communities there is an increase in the number of people with high blood pressure [5]. He was able to show a linear relationship between sodium intake and

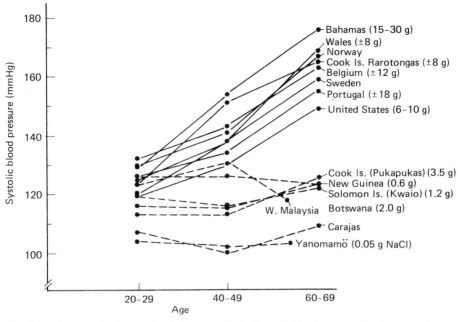

Fig. 5.1. Comparative international data on salt intake and blood pressure levels at varying ages. (Adapted from Joossens; see [2].) Values are averages for the two sexes. *Broken lines* indicate that no salt is added to food, *continuous lines* that salt is added.

blood pressure, with an increase of approximately 100 mmol/day of sodium in the diet causing an average increase in systolic and diastolic pressure of 12 mmHg and 7 mmHg respectively.

This sort of relationship does not, of course, necessarily imply causality. It is possible that there is some other factor in the diet which is in itself related to salt intake that may account for this relationship. At the present time a large, well-controlled

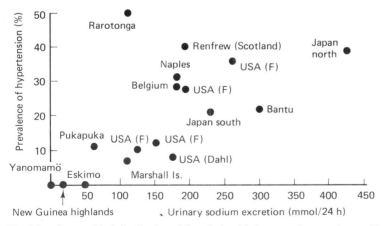

Fig. 5.2. Geographical distribution of the relationship between the prevalence of hypertension and 24-hour urinary sodium excretion. (See [4].)

multicentre study is being carried out to see whether, when studies are done prospectively and under similar controlled conditions, the same relationships are found between sodium excretion in the urine and blood pressure.

In general, when single populations have been studied, no relationship has been found between sodium excretion and blood pressure. This finding could be due to several factors. Firstly, as Simpson has pointed out [5], the range of salt intake in most Western communities is quite narrow, only varying from 100 to 200 mmol/day. In many individuals salt intake may vary from day to day by a similar amount. The measurement of 24-hour urinary sodium excretion in a group will reflect quite accurately the average intake for that population, but will not be so useful in characterising a particular individual's salt intake. Indeed some studies have claimed that only when 11 consecutive 24-hour urinary sodiums are collected can an accurate assessment of salt intake be made for that individual. Any relationship between salt intake and blood pressure in a single community would also be obscured by differences in susceptibility to the effect of salt. Nevertheless, when communities have been studied where there is a wider range of salt intake and each individual's salt intake is more consistent from day to day, direct relations have been shown between 24-hour urinary sodium excretion and blood pressure. Such communities include Korea [6], Japan [7] and, more recently, Kashmir [8].

Intervention Studies

Several studies where salt intake has been altered over a period of time do suggest that it could play a role in determining blood pressure levels within a community, although, as with much of the epidemiological evidence, the studies are not as well controlled as one would like. The best-controlled study is that of Hofman and colleagues from Holland [9], who randomised just under 500 newborn babies into two groups, one of which was placed on a restricted salt diet while the other group had a normal sodium intake. The study was double blind. In other words neither the mothers nor the investigators who were measuring the blood pressure knew which salt intake the baby was consuming. These babies were followed up over a period of 6 months, the difference in diet being maintained for this time. Spot urine checks showed that the urinary sodium concentration was reduced in the restricted salt intake group compared with the normal salt group. Over the 6 months of the follow-up there was a gradual and progressively increasing difference in systolic blood pressure, so that, by the end of 6 months, the babies with the restricted salt intake had a systolic pressure 2.1 mmHg lower than those on the usual salt intake ($p<0.01$). At this time the difference in diets was discontinued, so it is unclear what would have happened if the babies had continued with the difference in salt intake for a longer period of time.

Even if salt restriction only produced a 2-mmHg difference in blood pressure in adults over a long period of time, Rose has suggested that such a shift of the whole population's blood pressure downwards by this amount would considerably reduce cardiovascular risk, and the benefit derived would be similar to that of all of the current blood pressure lowering treatment being given to patients with established hypertension [10].

There have been intervention studies in adults, usually by chance rather than as a deliberate study. For instance, Samburu soldiers in the Kenyan army were given a large daily salt ration. With this increase in salt intake there was an increase in blood pressure, and at least part of this rise in blood pressure was attributed to the increase in salt intake [11]. Also in Africa, a rural tribe has been studied some of whose members migrated to a city. An increase in blood pressure was found in the migrants that was attributed at least in part to a difference in the dietary intake between the rural community and the urban community, particularly an increase in sodium intake and a reduction in potassium intake [12].

In two countries where salt intake has historically been very high, there have been government campaigns to try and reduce it. In Belgium it has fallen from its very high level in the 1950s of 15 g/day to approximately 9 g/day currently [13]. Similarly in Japan, where salt intake was estimated to average 14.5 g/day, it has now fallen to 12.5 g/day [14]. In both countries there has been a decrease in stroke mortality and a fall in the prevalence of high blood pressure [13,15]. It is not possible to ascertain from this type of study whether these two findings are causally related, and the results are complicated by the fact that stroke mortality has fallen in most Western countries over the last 50 to 100 years. Joossens [16] has suggested that this fall in stroke mortality may be related to a reduction in salt consumption in many Western countries over the same period, although there may be many other factors. As already mentioned, salt consumption probably reached its peak (around 300–500 mmol/day) in the late nineteenth century, when it was relatively very cheap and food consumed during the winter was preserved in it. With the advent of the refrigerator and the deep freeze, it is no longer necessary to preserve food in salt, and salt intake has fallen.

Lowering salt intake in a predominantly adult population may be less effective than if it is started early in life. Careful observation of those countries which are successful in reducing sodium intake may retrospectively provide the evidence to justify this change.

It is important to realise that it is unlikely that there will ever be definitive evidence, and recommendations that the whole population should reduce salt intake are based on the expectation that it may be beneficial and is unlikely to be harmful. At the very least it is generally agreed that salt intake should not be increased from the present levels.

Evidence in Animals other than Man

Meneely et al. [18] showed many years ago that in laboratory rats blood pressure at 9 months varied with the amount of salt in the diet (Fig. 5.3). An increase in salt intake has also been shown to cause a rise in blood pressure in normal baboons [19] and sheep [20]. Grollman [21] demonstrated that an increase in salt intake in normal pregnant rats resulted in their offspring having higher blood pressures that the offspring of pregnant rats given less sodium.

Dahl [22], by selective in-breeding of rats over five to seven generations, produced strains of rats which were either highly susceptible or resistant to salt, so that the susceptible rats developed severe hypertension when exposed to it. In a series of studies they demonstrated that if the rats were exposed to salt early in life they were then much more sensitive to sodium later in life. They also demonstrated that feeding the salt-sensitive rats the then available high-solute commerical baby food induced severe hypertension and increased mortality [23]. Parabiotic experiments, in which

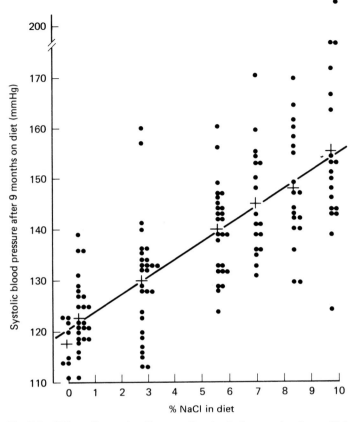

Fig. 5.3.   Effect of increasing dietary sodium intake in normal male rats (Adapted from [18].)

the two different strains of rats were grafted together, showed that the salt-resistant rat also had a rise in blood pressure in this situation, demonstrating that at least part of the rise in blood pressure was related to a humoral factor [24]. Further studies in which the kidneys were cross-transplanted between the two different strains of rats before they had developed high blood pressure, demonstrated that the kidney carried the message for the high blood pressure [25]. Subsequently Tobian showed that the kidney of the salt-sensitive rat, before the animal developed high blood pressure, was less able to excrete sodium than the kidney of the salt-resistant rat, and suggested that the genetic abnormality in the kidney of the Dahl rat was a difficulty in excreting sodium [26].

Studies in other strains of rats with inherited hypertension have also shown that blood pressure is increased when salt intake is increased, and in particular in one strain of rat the animals go through a phase when young during which they are much more sensitive to the effects of salt [27]. Cross-transplantation of the kidney between this and another strain of hypertensive rat has also demonstrated that the kidney is responsible for the high blood pressure [28,29]. Nearly all forms of experimental hypertension in rats and in other animals are made worse by a high salt intake [30].

Possible Mechanisms for Salt-induced Hypertension

In the early 1960s, before the demonstration that the kidney carried the message for the high blood pressure in the inherited forms of hypertension in rats, it was already being suggested that in humans with essential hypertension there might be a primary abnormality of the kidney causing sodium and water retention. This would give rise to an increasing amount of fluid in the extracellular space, and an increase in plasma volume, that would cause a rise in cardiac output. The greater the salt intake the greater the increase in plasma volume. It was thought that subsequently peripheral vascular resistance would increase by autoregulatory mechanisms, and in this way blood pressure would rise. At this stage negative feedback would reduce cardiac output towards normal and the raised blood pressure would cause the kidney to excrete more sodium. The high blood pressure would then cause further structural thickening of the small arterioles, giving rise to further narrowing and to a vicious cycle in the development of hypertension.

This concept has the disadvantage that no one has been able to demonstrate any evidence of plasma or extracellular fluid expansion in the early phase of hypertension. However, more recent evidence in man does suggest that the kidney may be responsible for the high blood pressure. For instance, studies of renal transplant recipients have shown that the donor's family history of hypertension appears to play an important role in determining the subsequent blood pressure in the recipient [31], and other studies have shown that, in patients who develop renal failure secondary to essential hypertension without malignant hypertension, kidney transplantation cures their high blood pressure [32].

Dahl first proposed in 1969 that, in his salt-sensitive rats, the rise in blood pressure could possibly be due to an increase in a sodium-excreting hormone, which was raised in order to try to get rid of the excess sodium, and, as a side effect, caused a rise in blood pressure [24]. These concepts were further developed by Haddy and Overbeck [33] and Blaustein [34] regarding volume-expanded hypertension, and man with essential hypertension. Blaustein was the first to point out a possible mechanism whereby a rise in intracellular sodium could, through inhibition of sodium–calcium exchange, cause a rise in intracellular calcium and thereby vascular reactivity [35]. de Wardener and MacGregor then suggested that patients with essential hypertension might, as in the Dahl rat, inherit a kidney that is less able to excrete sodium, and postulated that most forms of hypertension, whether primary or secondary, were due to normal volume control mechanisms correcting a persistent, inherited or acquired difficulty in excreting sodium [35]. These normal volume control mechanisms have as yet to be fully elucidated, but could include an increase in the secretion of the atrial natriuretic peptides and a postulated hypothalamic sodium transport inhibitor. The level of these hormones in the plasma and, with time, the severity of the blood pressure, would depend on the extent of the defect in the kidney's ability to excrete sodium and the salt intake. There is now some evidence that supports parts of these concepts, but there is still much controversy about the exact mechanisms involved. However, there is a considerable amount of evidence suggesting that there are abnormalities of sodium metabolism, particularly sodium transport across cell membranes, in many patients with essential hypertension.

Abnormalities of Sodium Metabolism in Human Hypertension

Several different abnormalities of sodium transport have now been described in the red blood cells of patients with essential hypertension [36]. Much more consistent results have been obtained in studies in white cells, where patients with hypertension have been shown to have an increase in white cell sodium concentration that appears to be related to a reduction in the ouabain-sensitive component of the sodium pump [37]. Further studies have shown that this inhibition of sodium transport across the white cell membrane is due to an increased level of an inhibitor in the plasma of patients with essential hypertension, and that the degree of inhibition is related to the severity of the hypertension [38]. Other studies, where the sodium transport inhibitor has been measured directly on biochemical or cytochemical bioassays, have also suggested that there may be a raised level of sodium transport inhibitor in patients with essential hypertension, and that that rise in the sodium transport inhibitor is related to the severity of the blood pressure, and in normal subjects in some studies is related to the salt intake [36].

To this may be added the recent characterisation and synthesis of the atrial natriuretic peptides, and the finding that they are potentially an important natriuretic hormone [37]. The plasma level is related to salt intake, and it was of interest to find that it is raised in patients with essential hypertension [39]. The reason for this rise is not fully understood, but one possible explanation could be an inherited or acquired defect in the kidney's ability to excrete sodium. Clearly much more work needs to be done to elucidate the mechanisms of the rise in blood pressure in essential hypertension, and particularly how this may relate to salt intake. It could well be that an understanding of the mechanism might obviate the need for further epidemiological evidence, which in any case is unlikely to be any more definitive than the evidence we have so far.

Should the Whole Population Cut its Salt Intake?

As can be seen from the above, much circumstantial and some direct evidence links salt intake to the development of high blood pressure. Nevertheless, some people are not convinced by this evidence, claiming that more direct evidence is required, and that it may be unwise for the whole population to cut back on its salt intake moderately. No harm appears to result from reducing salt intake moderately, and most Western health agencies and governments are now recommending that the whole population should do so.

A separate question which is not directly related to the epidemiological arguments is whether salt restriction lowers blood pressure when blood pressure is raised. Evidence for this is much easier to obtain, and more definitive answers can be given. Some have argued that since 10%–20% of the population may have high blood pressure, while by the age of 65–74 more than 65% of people in the United States and probably in other countries have definite or borderline hypertension, the public in general might benefit from a reduction in sodium intake, even though some persons do not presently require it.

Salt Restriction in Patients with High Blood Pressure

Many early studies clearly showed that the restriction of sodium intake to approximately the same level as that during evolution, about 1–20 mmol/day, caused a substantial fall in blood pressure in subjects with severe or malignant hypertension [40–42]. This was accompanied by a decrease in morbidity and mortality, with no adverse effects, except in subjects with pre-existing severe renal failure [42]. The diet as usually prescribed was very monotonous, and many patients had difficulty in sticking to it for long periods of time. Therefore, with the advent of diuretics and other drugs to lower blood pressure, in the late 1950s, severe salt restriction was abandoned as a routine way of treating hypertension. More recent evidence has shown that less

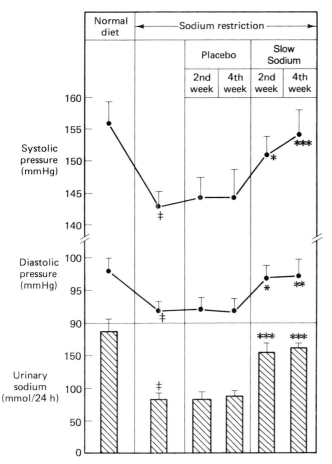

Fig. 5.4. Systolic and diastolic blood pressure and 24-hour urinary sodium excretion in 19 patients studied on their normal diet, 2 weeks after dietary sodium restriction (approx. 80 mmol/day) and at 2-weekly intervals during a randomised crossover trial of Slow Sodium tablets versus placebo. Error bars are ± sem. ***$p<0.001$; **$p<0.01$; *$p<0.05$ comparing measurements on Slow Sodium with placebo. ‡$p<0.001$ comparing measurement on normal diet with 2 weeks of dietary sodium restriction. (From [44], with kind permission of the *Lancet*.)

severe restriction of sodium intake, to about 80 mmol/day, can also cause a fall in blood pressure [43–45], even in patients with mild to moderate hypertension (Fig. 5.4); perhaps more importantly, the effect of sodium restriction is in addition to that of other blood pressure lowering drugs [46–48]. On the other hand, it has been known for many years that short-term reduction in sodium intake in subjects with normal blood pressure has little effect in reducing it. This finding led to some confusion when some studies on restricting salt intake in patients with borderline or normal blood pressure found no effect. The authors then claimed that their results applied to people with more severe hypertension [49].

The mechanism for this different response to salt restriction between normotensive and hypertensive subjects has now been shown to be due largely to a diminished response of the renin–angiotensin system to salt restriction in subjects with hypertension. In other words, when normal subjects reduce sodium intake there is a rise in the release of renin and formation of angiotensin II, a powerful vasoconstrictor, which largely prevents the blood pressure fall that would have occurred. However, in many patients with essential hypertension there is a reduced rise in renin, and less angiotensin II is formed, and the blood pressure falls. This concept has been confirmed, both from measurements of the components of the renin–angiotensin system during salt restriction, and by the use of saralasin [50], a competitive inhibitor of angiotensin II. More recently the angiotensin-converting enzyme inhibitors that block the formation of angiotensin I from angiotensin II have also been used. Whilst the evidence that sodium restriction lowers blood pressure is mainly based on short-term trials, and although there is no doubt that longer term, better controlled studies are needed, particularly in combination with other non-pharmacological methods and/or drug treatment, it makes sense in the light of present knowledge to instruct patients to restrict their salt intake moderately, as well as to give them other non-pharmacological advice on lowering their blood pressure. If this does not control the blood pressure, which it may not in many patients, particularly those with more severe hypertension, the addition of a converting enzyme inhibitor or a beta blocker will be a particularly effective combination, often avoiding the need for diuretic therapy. Indeed, much circumstantial evidence suggests that salt restriction is as effective as a diuretic in the treatment of hypertension, without the latter's metabolic side effects.

How Practical is Moderate Salt Restriction?

Only 5%–10% of our present sodium consumption occurs naturally in food. In other words, the great majority of the salt we eat is added to food either during processing, during cooking or at the table. If the diet was restricted to fresh meat, fresh fish, fruit and vegetables, and cereals without added salt, we would be on what is now considered to be a very low sodium diet, but in fact would only be equivalent to the salt intake of our early ancestors. More and more of the food that we eat has been processed, and during this processing salt is added. Nevertheless, in our experience and that of Simpson [51], most subjects have little difficulty in reducing salt intake to around 70–80 mmol/day. This would halve present consumption, and could be done by not adding salt to food at the table or during cooking and by avoiding food known to have a high sodium content.

Adaptation to changes in sodium intake occur quite quickly, with increased sensitivity of the salt taste receptors allowing detection of salt in food where it was not previously detectable. This normally takes around 3–6 weeks. Often subjects then notice that the high-salt foods they used to like taste very unpleasant. Simpson has pointed out that sodium restriction of this order is much easier to achieve than getting subjects to lose weight or to reduce their alcohol consumption. However, there is an unresolved difficulty for people who wish to restrict sodium intake but have to eat away from home, as it is then very difficult to discover the sodium content of the food being consumed and usually it is very high. Clearly the labelling of processed food with its sodium content would be of great help to those who wish to reduce salt intake but want to have the convenience of such foods.

The high sodium content of dried cow's milk and other out-dated baby foods has already been recognised and the levels in these foods have been much reduced. However, there is evidence that sodium intake is rising in children with the increased advertising and consumption of high-sodium snacks and processed foods [51]. This is of particular concern as it may make these children more susceptible to the development of hypertension later in life. The food industry could help by producing snack foods that contain less sodium. There is no evidence that this would make them less acceptable. Even Simpson, who was previously sceptical about the effects of sodium restriction, finds it a curious reflection on our present dietary customs that a 30-gram can of chocolate pudding contains 1% sodium chloride [52].

One major difficulty in reducing sodium intake is the salt content of bread, which contributes substantially to the salt intake of most people in the United Kingdom. A gradual reduction in the salt content of bread would perhaps be one of the easiest ways of reducing sodium intake. It is interesting in this regard to reflect that in certain areas of Italy, where salt taxes were historically very high, the use of salt in bread was stopped. These areas still have salt-free bread, showing once again that the salt content of food is merely a habit which can be changed by historical accident.

Other Dietary Factors and Blood Pressure

Whilst most studies relating blood pressure to diet have in the past concentrated on salt intake, there is increasing evidence that other constituents of the diet may have an important influence.

The most impressive evidence so far concerns potassium. Epidemiological studies have shown a positive correlation of urinary sodium : potassium ratio and plasma potassium with blood pressure, and a negative correlation with potassium excretion [53]. Studies in which potassium chloride has been added to the diet, roughly doubling potassium intake, have shown a fall in blood pressure in hypertensive subjects [54] but little change in normotensives [55]. Animal studies and one epidemiological study in man have suggested that increasing potassium intake may protect from stroke, independently of the effect on blood pressure [56].

Calcium intake has been claimed to be related to blood pressure [57], but re-analysis of the data has shown this to be unlikely, or to be confounded by other variables [58]. Similarly, claims that calcium supplementation of the diet may lower blood pressure have not been substantiated, although it is possible that some subgroups might react in this way [59].

Studies in animals have suggested that magnesium intake may influence blood pressure, but studies in man are lacking. However, one well-controlled study of magnesium supplementation failed to show any fall in blood pressure in established hypertensives [60].

Some studies have suggested that reducing saturated fat intake may have a lowering effect on blood pressure [61], but controlled studies in which the diet has been supplemented with polyunsaturated fats have shown little change. A vegetarian diet has also been shown to lower blood pressure, but it is not clear what factor in the diet is responsible [62]. Increases in fibre intake may lower blood pressure, but further work is needed.

Epidemiological studies have clearly shown that alcohol intake is related to blood pressure [63], and some have suggested that reducing alcohol intake may lower it. Current advice suggests alcohol intake should not exceed 2–3 units/day.

Weight, and therefore obesity, are closely related to blood pressure. However, some recent studies suggest that high blood pressure in obese individuals carries less risk than in the lean (64–66).

It therefore makes sense, in patients with high blood pressure and perhaps in the whole population, that if they are going to reduce salt intake, they should reduce saturated fat intake, and eat more fresh fruit and vegetables, as this will increase potassium as well as fibre intake; these measures in themselves may lower blood pressure and could also independently reduce the risk of vascular disease.

Summary

There is much circumstantial and some direct evidence to suggest that a high consumption of salt may predispose individuals and communities to the development of high blood pressure. However, studies to prove a definite causative relationship are unlikely to be done, for the practical reason that they would need to be carried out over a whole generation.

Short-term reduction of salt intake lowers blood pressure in many subjects with established hypertension, but has little effect in subjects with normal blood pressure.

Recommendations for the whole population to reduce salt intake are therefore based on the expectation that it may reduce the prevalence of high blood pressure in the community, and is unlikely to be harmful. Those with known high blood pressure should be advised to reduce salt intake, as this may lower it and is additive to the effect of blood-pressure-reducing drugs.

Other dietary factors, particularly potassium intake, may also be of importance in influencing blood pressure.

References

1. Denton D (1982) The hunger for salt. An anthropological, physiological and medical analysis. Springer, Berlin Heidelberg New York
2. Oliver WJ, Cohen EL, Neel JV (1975) Blood pressure, sodium intake and sodium-related hormones in the Yanomamo Indians, a "no-salt culture". Circulation 52:146–151

3. Joossens JV (1980) Dietary salt restriction: the case in favour. The therapeutics of hypertension. Royal Society of Medicine, London, pp 243–250 (International congress and symposium series 26)
4. MacGregor GA (1985) Sodium is more important than calcium in essential hypertension. Hypertension 7:628–637
5. Simpson FO (1984) Salt and hypertension: current data, attitudes and policies. J Cardiovasc Pharmacol 6:S4–S9
6. Kesteloot H, Park BC, Lee CS, Brems-Heyns E, Joossens JV (1980) A comparative study of blood pressure and sodium intake in Belgium and in Korea. In: Kesteloot H, Joossens JV (eds) Epidemiology of arterial blood pressure. Martinus Nijhoff, The Hague, pp 453–470
7. Yamori Y, Kihara M, Nara Y et al. (1981) Hypertension and diet: multiple regression analysis in a Japanese farming community. Lancet I:120
8. Mir MA, Mir F, Khosla T (1984) High incidence of hypertension in heavy salt consuming population of northern Kashmir. Circulation 70 (suppl II):359 (abstract)
9. Hofman A, Hazebroek A, Volkenburg HA (1983) A randomised trial of sodium intake and blood pressure in newborn infants. JAMA 250:370–373
10. Rose G (1981) Strategy of prevention: lessons from cardiovascular disease. Br Med J 282:1847–1851
11. Shaper AG, Leonard PJ, Jones KW, Jones M (1969) Environmental effects on the body build, blood pressure and blood chemistry of nomadic warriors serving in the army of Kenya. East Afr Med J 46:282–289
12. Poulter N, Khaw KT, Hopwood BEC, Mugambi M, Peart WS, Sever PS (1984) Salt and blood pressure in various populations. J Cardiovasc Pharmacol 6:S197–S203
13. Joossens JV, Geboers J (1983) Salt and hypertension. Prev Med 12:53–59
14. National nutritional survey (1981) Ministry of Health and Welfare, Koseisho, Japan
15. National survey on circulatory disorders (1980) Ministry of Health and Welfare, Koseisho, Japan
16. Joossens JV, Kesteloot H, Amery A (1979) Salt intake and mortality from stroke. N Engl J Med 300:1396
17. Longmate N (1966) King cholera – the biography of a disease. Hamish Hamilton, London
18. Ball COT, Meneely GR (1957) Observations on dietary sodium chloride. J Am Diet Assoc 33:366–370
19. Cherchovich GM, Capek K, Jefremova Z, Pohlova I, Jelinek J (1976) High salt intake and blood pressure in lower primates. J Appl Physiol 40:601–604
20. Whitworth JA, Coghlan JP, Denton DA, Hardy K, Scoggins BA (1979) Effect of sodium loading and ACTH on blood pressure of sheep with reduced renal mass. Cardiovasc Res 13:9–15
21. Grollman A, Grollman EF (1962) The teratogenic induction of hypertension. J Clin Invest 41:710–714
22. Knudsen KD, Dahl LK (1966) Essential hypertension: inborn error of sodium metabolism. Postgrad Med J 42:148–152
23. Dahl LK, Heine N, Leitl G, Tassinari L (1970) Hypertension and death from consumption of processed baby foods in rats. Proc Soc Exp Biol Med 133:1405–1408
24. Dahl LK, Knudsen KD, Iwai J (1969) Humoral transmission of hypertension: evidence from parabiosis. Circ Res 25:21–33
25. Dahl LK, Heine N (1975) Primary role of renal homographs in setting chronic blood pressure levels in rats. Circ Res 36:692–696
26. Tobian L, Lange J, Azei S et al. (1978) Reduction of natriuretic capacity in renin release in isolated blood perfused kidneys of Dahl hypertension-prone rats. Circ Res 43(Suppl I):92–97
27. Aoki K, Yamori Y, Ooshim A (1972) Effects of high or low sodium intake in spontaneously hypertensive rats. Jpn Circ J 36:539
28. Bianchi G, Fox U, Di Francesco GF, Giovanetti AM, Pagetti D (1974) Blood pressure changes by kidney cross-transplantation between spontaneously hypertensive rats and normotensive rats. Clin Sci Mol Med 47:435–438
29. Kawabe K, Watanabe TX, Shiono K, Sokabe H (1979) Influence of blood pressure on renal isographs between spontaneously hypertensive and normotensive rats utilizing the F1 hybrids. Jpn Heart J 20:886–894
30. Haddy FJ (1980) Mechanism, prevention and therapy of sodium dependent hypertension. Am J Med 69:746–758
31. Guidi C, Avanzi C, Bianchi G (1984) Familial factors in hypertension after renal transplantation (abstract). Proceedings of IXth international congress of nephrology, Los Angeles, California, 1984, p 209
32. Curtis JJ, Luke RG, Dustan HP et al. (1983) Remission of essential hypertension after renal transplantation. N Engl J Med 309:1009–1015
33. Haddy FJ, Overbeck HW (1976) The role of humoral agents in volume expanded hypertension. Life Sci 19:935–948

34. Blaustein MP (1977) Sodium ions, calcium ions, blood pressure regulation and hypertension: a reassessment and a hypothesis. Am J Physiol 232:C165–C173

35. de Wardener HE, MacGregor GA (1980) Dahl's hypothesis that a saluretic substance may be responsible for a sustained rise in arterial pressure: its possible role in essential hypertension. Kidney Int 18:1–9

36. de Wardener HE, MacGregror GA (1983) The relation to a circulating transport inhibitor (the natriuretic hormone?) to hypertension. Medicine 62:310–326

37. Hilton PJ (1986) Cellular sodium transport in essential hypertension. N Engl J Med 314:222–229

38. Gray HH, Hilton PJ, Richardson PJ (1986) Effect of serum from patients with essential hypertension on sodium transport in normal leucocytes. Clin Sci 70:583–586

39. Sagnella GA, Markandu ND, Shore AC, MacGregor GA (1986) Raised circulating levels of atrial natriuretic peptides in essential hypertension. Lancet I:179–181

40. Ambard L, Beaujard E (1904) Causes de l'hypertension arterielle. Arch Gen Med I:520–533

41. Allen FM, Sherrill JW (1922) The treatment of arterial hypertension. J Metab Res 2:429–546

42. Kempner W (1948) Treatment of hypertensive vascular disease with rice diet. Am J Med 4:545–577

43. Parijs J, Joossens JV, Van der Linden L, Verstreken G, Amery AKPC (1973) Moderate sodium restriction and diuretics in the treatment of hypertension. Am Heart J 85:22–34

44. Morgan T, Adams W, Gillies A, Wilson M, Morgan G, Carney S (1978) Hypertension treated by salt restriction. Lancet I:227–230

45. MacGregor GA, Markandu ND, Best FE, et al. (1982) Double blind randomised crossover trial of moderate sodium restriction in essential hypertension. Lancet I:351–356

46. Beard TC, Cooke HM, Gray WR, Barge R (1982) Randomised controlled trial of a no-added sodium diet for mild hypertension. Lancet II:455–458

47. Erwteman TM, Nagelkerke N, Lubsen J, Kouta M, Dunning AJ (1984) Beta-blockade, diuretics and salt restriction for the management of mild hypertension: a randomised double blind trial. Br Med J 289:406–409

48. MacGregor GA, Markandu ND, Singer DRJ, Cappuccio FP, Shore AC, Sagnella GA (1987) Moderate sodium restriction with angiotensin converting enzyme inhibitor in essential hypertension: a double blind study. Br Med J 294:531–534

49. Watt GCM, Edwards C, Hart JT, Hart M, Walton P, Foy CJW (1983) Dietary sodium restriction for mild hypertension in general practice. Br Med J 286:432–436

50. Cappuccio FP, Markandu ND, Sagnella GA, MacGregor GA (1985) Sodium restriction lowers high blood pressure through a decreased responsiveness of the renin system: direct evidence using saralasin. J Hypertens 3:243–247

51. De Courcy S, Mitchell H, Simmons D, MacGregor GA (1986) Urinary sodium excretion in 4–6 year old children: a cause for concern? Br Med J 292:1428–1429

52. Simpson FO (1982) Salt and hypertension. NZ Med J 95:420–421

53. MacGregor GA (1983) Dietary sodium and potassium intake and blood pressure. Lancet I:750–753

54. Khaw K-T, Thom S (1982) Randomised double-blind cross-over trial of potassium on blood pressure in normal subjects. Lancet II:1127–1129

55. MacGregor GA, Smith SJ, Markandu ND et al. (1982) Moderate potassium supplementation in essential hypertension. Lancet II:567

56. Khaw K-T, Barrett-Connor E (1987) Dietary potassium and stroke-associated mortality. N Engl J Med 316:235–240

57. McCarron DA, Morris ED, Henry HJ, Stanton JL (1984) Blood pressure and nutrient intake in the United States. Science 224:1392–1398

58. Feinleib N, Lenfant C, Miller SA (1984) Hypertension and calcium. Science 226:384–386

59. Grubbee DE, Hofman A (1986) Effect of calcium supplementation on diastolic blood pressure in young people with hypertension. Lancet II:703–706

60. Cappuccio FP, Markandu ND, Beynon GW, Shore AC, Sampson B, MacGregor GA (1985) Lack of effect of oral magnesium on high blood pressure: a double blind study. Br Med J 291:235–238

61. Puska P, Iacono JM, Nissinen A et al. (1983) Controlled, randomised trial of the effect of dietary fat on blood pressure. Lancet I:1–5

62. Rouse IL, Beilin LJ, Armstrong Bk, Vandongen R (1983) Blood-pressure-lowering effect of a vegetarian diet: controlled trial in normotensive subjects. Lancet I:5–10

63. Savdie E, Grosslight GM, Adena MA (1984) Relation of alcohol and cigarette consumption to blood pressure and serum creatinine levels. J Chron Dis 37:617–623

64. Barrett-Connor E, Khaw K-T (1985) Is hypertension more benign when associated with obesity? Circulation 72:53–60

65. Cambien F, Chretien JM, Ducimetiere P et al. (1985) Is the relationship between blood pressure and cardiovascular risk dependent on body mass index? Am J Epidemiol 122:434–442

66. Elliot P, Shipley MJ, Rose G (1987) Are lean hypertensives at greater risk than obese hypertensives? J Hypertens 5(Suppl 5) S517–S519

Commentary

Rivers: I am concerned about the variability in the data in Fig. 5.3, and the fact that it has been presented so as to suggest a linear relationship between salt intake and blood pressure. I think that the variability of the data makes the line drawn rather arbitrary. A correlation coefficient may not be the right way to deal with such variability, given the clustering of the data along the *x*-axis.

Also, I am astounded that a 2 mmHg difference in blood pressure would considerably reduce cardiovascular risk for the population. It would seem to me important in making statements of this kind to define quite why the 2 mmHg drop in blood pressure occurred. Surely a mean drop of 2 mmHg due to a selective reduction in the blood pressure of that section of the population whose blood pressures were highest ought to be very different from a drop of 2 mmHg for everybody.

Sanders: The argument advanced by Rose (MacGregor's ref. 10) that a 2 mmHg reduction in the mean blood pressure would considerably reduce cardiovascular risk is extremely dubious. While the evidence for treatment of severe hypertension and reduction of risk of stroke is impressive, the evidence that treatment of mild hypertension is of benefit is equivocal. There is little evidence that normotensive subjects show a reduction in blood pressure from moderate sodium restriction. Therefore, it is illogical to advocate a reduction in salt intakes for the whole population. It is interesting to note that the incidence of stroke has fallen in the United Kingdom over the past 50 years. During this period there has been a shift away from traditionally preserved foods towards refrigerated foods. These preserved foods, besides having a relatively high salt content, also contained high concentrations of several other compounds such as tyramine and histamine that could increase blood pressure.

Some caucasian vegetarian populations seem to have lower blood pressures than the omnivorous population, but this is not the case in the United Kingdom or for Indian vegetarians. Vegetarians tend to be lighter in weight than average, and some groups may have a more relaxed lifestyle (e.g. Zen macrobiotic vegetarians and Seventh-day Adventist vegetarians). Caution therefore has to be exercised before suggesting that a vegetarian diet has a specific blood-pressure-lowering attribute.

While I agree that moderate sodium restriction can easily be implemented, I am not convinced by the argument that the sodium intake of the general population should be reduced because such a reduction apparently does no harm. If it spoils enjoyment of food it certainly does harm. On the other hand, it is quite reasonable to caution against further increasing salt intakes on two grounds: firstly it might raise blood pressure, and secondly it might increase the risk of stomach cancer.

Durnin: In discussing whether the whole population should cut its salt intake. MacGregor says that "some people are not convinced by this evidence". To my knowledge, many leading authorities on hypertension are quite sceptical about the relationship between salt intake and hypertension, yet almost no mention is made of these contrary views.

Curzon: Concerning the use of salt in the diet there seems to be one fundamental problem in any endeavour to restrict salt intake in Western cultures. There is much evidence that in countries such as the United Kingdom or United States the average person eats six or seven times per day. However, of greater importance is that 20% of meals are eaten away from the home. This is mentioned, but nevertheless it is very difficult for a person to find foods low in salt when eating in restaurants. Many such foods contain substantial quantities of salt and some foods, such as Chinese, are notoriously salty.

Short of a diet restricted to natural fruits and vegetables, there are very few opportunities to eat a low salt diet. In practice achieving low salt intake is difficult, and the problem is not fully addressed in the paper.

Chapter 6

Dietary Fat and Coronary Heart Disease

T. A. B. Sanders

Introduction

Coronary heart disease (CHD) is a major public health problem because a high proportion of its victims are middle-aged men: an apparently healthy man in his fifties can leave home for work in the morning and be dead an hour later, his wife a widow without support. Women, at least before the menopause, are less prone to the disease than men. It is estimated that about 1 in 5 men suffer a heart attack before the age of 65 and a high proportion of attacks are fatal. However, the average age of death from CHD is 74 years [1]. The individual is concerned about whether he will live longer and whether he will have less disability, not about what is written on his death certificate. As immortality is not an alternative, sudden death from CHD in the geriatric population has advantages over other causes of death such as stroke and cancer, which involve more suffering and an increased burden on society. The aim perhaps should be to defer rather than prevent CHD. Dietary fat has been implicated in the causation of CHD, and changes in fat intake have been recommended for the general population. This article critically reviews the available evidence.

Epidemiology

CHD mortality rates for men aged 45–64 are highest in North America, northern Europe and Australasia, where most of the dietary fat is derived from meat and dairy products [2,3]. The mortality rates from CHD are low in Japan and in Greenland Eskimos [4], although death rates from other forms of cardiovascular disease such as stroke are greater. It is generally held that CHD rates are low in many developing countries, but reliable mortality statistics are not available. Mortality rates appear to be intermediate in southern Mediterranean countries, where olive oil is the main source of dietary fat. There are several anomalies in the data. For example France, a country with a similar fat intake to other northern European countries, appears to have very low rates of CHD. This might be due to difference in death certification, as total mortality rates are similar to those in other European countries. However,

French immigrants to the United Kingdom have lower CHD rates than the indigenous population [5]. CHD mortality rates are higher in Indian men of Asian descent in Great Britain than in the indigenous population [5]. Yet their diet conforms in many respects to that advocated by the British Department of Health and Social Security [1]. A high incidence of CHD is found among Indian men in other parts of the world [6] as well as in urban India. The popular view that CHD is a disease of affluence seems incorrect as mortality rates are highest in the least affluent areas of the United Kingdom and in the lowest socioeconomic classes [7]. CHD mortality rates in 45–65-year-old men are highest in Scotland, Northern Ireland and South Wales. Irish and Scottish immigrants to England also have higher than average rates of cardiovascular mortality.

Changes in CHD mortality have occurred in several countries over the past 20–30 years [1,2]. Most notable is the decline in CHD rates in women which has occurred in 26 countries. It is particularly marked in all areas of the United Kingdom and is in contrast to the trend in men, which was upwards but now may be falling. Over the past decade CHD mortality has decreased in the United States, Finland and Australia; no change in total fat intake has occurred in these countries but there may have been changes in the types of fats consumed. CHD rates have also been declining in Japan, both in men and in women, despite massive industrialisation. Countries showing increases in CHD rates are Sweden, Poland, Czechoslovakia, Northern Ireland and Hungary.

Transmigration studies of populations migrating from an area of low incidence of CHD to one of high incidence suggest that the disease pattern is acquired on migration. For example, Japanese in Hawaii and in California have similar rates of CHD to the indigenous population [8]. Migration in the opposite direction to areas where the incidence is low has been accompanied by a decreased risk of CHD. For example, the incidence of CHD in second-generation Jewish immigrants to Israel is lower than in New York [9].

Risk Factors

Large-scale prospective studies have led to the identification of risk factors for CHD. High blood pressure, cigarette smoking and high serum cholesterol were found to be independent predictors of death from CHD. A combination of risk factors amplified the risk of CHD [10]. Diet has not emerged as a good predictor of risk in prospective studies. The prevalence of hypertension and frequency of cigarette smoking is greater in Japanese men than in Europeans, but serum cholesterol concentrations are low and their incidence of CHD is low. This led to the view that a high plasma cholesterol concentration was a prerequisite for CHD. However, there are populations with relatively low serum cholesterol concentrations and high CHD rates. For example Asian men of Indian descent have a greatly increased risk of CHD that is not explained by these traditional risk factors [6].

Attempts have been made using multivariate analysis to quantify the risk. These studies show that heredity is the best predictor of risk [11], followed by cigarette smoking. Smoking is almost certainly the over-riding cause of CHD in men aged less than 45 or 50 [12].

An elevated serum cholesterol concentration in the absence of other risk factors is not a particularly powerful predictor of risk. Moreover, CHD rates may vary threefold in populations with similar serum cholesterol concentrations [13]. Most of the plasma cholesterol is carried by low density lipoproteins (LDL), and elevations of both total and LDL cholesterol are positively correlated with CHD. The risk of developing CHD is proportional to the initial plasma total cholesterol concentration in men aged 30–62 years and in women up to the age 50 years [10]. However, the predictive power of plasma total cholesterol concentration for CHD decreases with age. The Lipid Research Clinics Pooling Project suggested that there was a curvilinear relationship between serum cholesterol and risk of CHD (Fig. 6.1). The threshold concentration above which risk increased was 200–220 mg/100 ml [14]. Plasma cholesterol concentrations are low, about 150 mg/100 ml, until the age of 25 years and they subsequently increase with age until about 40 years of age, when about half the adult population have cholesterol concentrations in excess of 200 mg/100 ml (Fig. 6.2). A high proportion of those who die from CHD have plasma cholesterol concentrations below 200 mg/100 ml. This has been interpreted by some commentators as meaning that the relationship between plasma cholesterol and CHD risk is linear.

Serum triglyceride concentration emerged as a risk factor in prospective studies using univariate analysis, but not with multivariate analysis [15]. Obesity has not emerged as an independent risk factor. The pattern of fat deposition, on the other hand, is a better predictor of risk, particularly upper body obesity, which is reflected in the waist : hip ratio [16]. The pattern of fat distribution is not correlated with the intake of any specific nutrient or the proportion of energy derived from fat. Non-insulin-dependent diabetes mellitus (NIDDM) is a risk factor for CHD among some but not all populations. NIDDM is about four times more prevalent among Asian Indian

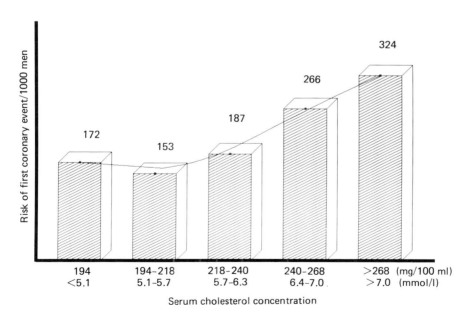

Fig. 6.1. Curvilinear relationship between the risk of coronary heart disease in men and serum cholesterol concentration. (Data taken from the Pooling Project Research Group [14].)

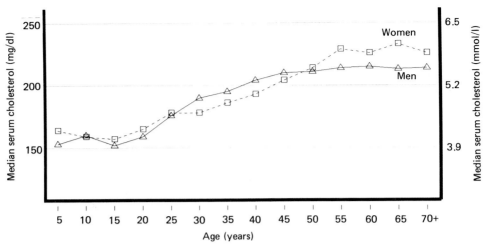

Fig. 6.2. Change in median serum cholesterol concentration with age in men and women. (Data from the *Lipid Research Clinics Population Studies Data Book*, vol 1. NIH publication 80–1527, US Government Printing Office, Washington, DC, 1980.)

men in the United Kingdom than in the general population [17]. This might explain their high incidence of CHD.

A negative correlation between high density lipoprotein (HDL) cholesterol concentration and coronary mortality has been a consistent finding within populations [18]. However, the mean HDL cholesterol concentrations appear to be high in populations with a high incidence of CHD, but low in those where it is rare. Within high-incidence populations that have high LDL levels, HDL and apolipoprotein A1 concentrations or the ratio of total to HDL cholesterol appear to be superior predictors of atherosclerosis in individual patients. In patients with hypertriglyceridaemia [19], LDL apolipoprotein B concentration is a better predictor of risk for coronary atherosclerosis than total or LDL cholesterol. It is noteworthy that low HDL concentrations are associated with NIDDM and hyperinsulinaemia [20]. More recently fibrinogen and clotting factor VII have been shown to be independent risk factors [21]. Cigarette smoking increases plasma fibrinogen concentrations and this might partly explain the relationship between smoking and CHD.

Pathology

CHD embraces a collection of several different disorders with related pathologies: myocardial infarction, angina pectoris and sudden cardiac death. Myocardial ischaemia is a common feature and results from an inadequate supply of oxygenated blood to the myocardium by the coronary arteries. This is either caused or exacerbated by coronary atherosclerosis. Coronary atherosclerosis is believed to develop slowly over 20 or 30 years or more. It would be predicted, therefore, that any dietary intervention adopted in middle life would be unlikely to have a marked impact on atherosclerosis. If dietary intervention is to be effective then it should begin at least in early adult life.

The human atherosclerotic lesion is a multi-layered matrix of fibrin, connective tissue and lipid. Atherosclerosis is associated with fibrin deposition, and more recent studies using new histochemical techniques for staining platelet-specific proteins such as β-thromboglobulin imply that blood platelets are involved in these early lesions. Ross [22] proposes that lesions occur in response to injury. Platelets, leucocytes and tissue macrophages are attracted to the site of injury. These cells release compounds that cause smooth muscle cells to proliferate, producing a raised gelatinous lesion. The lesion either heals or goes on to develop into a lipid-rich complex lesion. Because the first lesion that is easily visible macroscopically is the fatty streak in young children, it was assumed that this was the precursor of all types of lesion, including fibrous plaques. However, unlike the early proliferative gelatinous lesions, fatty streaks are not enriched in LDL. Smith [23] and other workers have argued that proliferation precedes lipid accumulation and that fatty streaks are irrelevant to the atherosclerotic process.

An assumption underlying much of the epidemiological study of CHD is that the clinical manifestations of CHD are largely, if not entirely, due to atheroma. Coronary atherosclerosis is present in most adults, but only a fraction, roughly one third, develop clinical CHD. The epidemiological characteristics of chronic vessel wall disease and clinical CHD are dissimilar. For example, the demonstration that risk of CHD from smoking is partly reversible, and is a short-term effect, is not consistent with a chronic disease and cannot logically be attributed to a decrease in the severity of atherosclerosis. This suggests that there must be another pathological process involved and this is likely to be thrombosis.

Post-mortem coronary angiographic studies show that coronary occlusion is most commonly caused by a blood clot (coronary thrombosis) resulting from the rupture of an atherosclerotic plaque. Coronary vasospasm [24] may also lead to coronary occlusion, although this is less common. Sudden cardiac death often results from ventricular fibrillation. Indeed, the pathology of CHD implies that several factors interact to produce the disease: the generation of the lesion, and haemostatic variables such as blood pressure, blood viscosity, cellular components and the coagulation and fibrinolytic pathways.

Epidemiological Associations of CHD with Fat Intake

International Comparisons

International comparisons show an association between fat consumption and CHD. This is seen most clearly when fat is expressed as a percentage of the calories. However, fat is a symbol of affluence, and may merely be acting as a marker of other aspects of Western lifestyle. There are, however, populations with a high proportion of energy derived from fat and a low incidence of CHD, for example Greenland Eskimos [25] and South Pacific Islanders [26]. A stronger correlation is found between saturated fatty acid intake, as a percentage of the energy intake, and CHD rates. Keys, in the Seven Countries study, showed that national percentage of energy derived from saturated fat was correlated with death from CHD and with serum cholesterol [13]. An extremely low incidence of CHD and atherosclerosis has also been observed in populations that eat large amounts of C20–22 polyunsaturated fatty acids derived from fish or marine mammals [27].

Intrapopulation Studies

In contrast to the between-country association, the relationship between saturated fat intake and risk of CHD within the general population of any particular country is either non-existent or very weak [28]. However, in Western countries the diet is relatively homogeneous with respect to the fatty acid composition of the dietary fat. Secondly, there are a number of difficulties in estimating the quality of fat intake owing to the variability in margarine composition, the variability in the fat content of meat and the lack of reliable data on processed foods. Prospective studies of diet are hard to interpret, as diet is a dynamic variable. Most studies have used a 24-hour dietary recall to estimate dietary intake. It is questionable whether one 24-hour dietary recall is representative of an individual's diet for the next 20 years.

Comparisons made between groups which have widely differing intakes of saturated fat compared with the average do, however, show a relationship between saturated fat intake and CHD. For example vegans, who consume no animal fats, and whose diets contain less than 10% saturated fat, do have a much lower incidence of CHD than lactovegetarians and meat-eaters [29].

In the Edinburgh–Stockholm study [30] a higher proportion of linoleic acid in adipose tissue was found in the Swedish men than in the Scottish men, and this correlated with a lower death rate from CHD. Subsequent studies in the Scottish population have revealed lower proportions of linoleic acid in patients with angina than in unaffected case controls [31]. However, the association between linoleic acid and CHD was confused by the observation that smokers have lower proportions of linoleic acid than controls. Using multivariate analysis it was shown that the proportion of linoleic acid in adipose tissue was independently related to risk of CHD in a dose-dependent manner. However, the range of linoleic acid in adipose tissue was small. The proportion of eicosapentaenoic acid in platelet lipids was also found to be negatively correlated with risk of CHD, but again the range encountered was small. It is difficult to perceive how such small differences could be biologically meaningful.

The level of linoleic acid in adipose tissue is held to be a good reflection of the dietary intake of linoleic acid. However, the proportion of linoleic acid that is incorporated into adipose tissue will also depend upon endogenous fatty acid production. For example, fatty acids of hepatic origin which are incorporated into very low density lipoprotein triglycerides can be delivered to adipose tissue. High proportions of linoleic acid have been reported in the adipose tissue and plasma phospholipids of strict vegetarians and these correlate with high intakes of linoleic acid [32] and a low CHD mortality rate. In contrast, higher proportions of linoleic acid are also found in the men of Indian descent who have a greater risk of CHD than the indigenous European population in the United Kingdom [33].

Thomas et al. [34] claimed that the level of *trans* fatty acids in adipose tissue was associated with the incidence of CHD in various regions of the United Kingdom. The work of Thomas has been strongly criticised on methodological grounds, because no allowance was made for other risk factors or for the differences in prosperity between the varying regions. Moreover, case-controlled studies have failed to show that patients with CHD have higher levels of *trans* fatty acids in their adipose tissue than those who are free from the disease.

Caucasian vegetarians have a lower risk of CHD under the age of 65 years than the general population [29,35]. However, as a group they tend not to smoke or drink alcohol excessively. CHD mortality rates were found to be similarly low among Seventh-day Adventist omnivores and lactovegetarians, but markedly lower among the vegan Seventh-day Adventists. Burr carried out a prospective study on the users of health food shops and found that CHD and total mortality rates were approximately half those in the general population. Even though the vegetarian users of the health food shops had lower rates of CHD than the omnivores this difference was not significant. A number of clinical studies have been carried out on vegetarians in order to explain their lower risk of CHD. Lower blood pressures, body weight, and percentage body fat have been reported [32,36]. Lower concentrations of vitamin-K-dependent clotting factors II, VII and X have also been noted in vegetarians [37]. Serum cholesterol concentrations tend to be similar in lactovegetarians compared with omnivores [38], but to be considerably lower in vegans [39]. While the fat intake of lactovegetarians and omnivores tends to be similar, that of vegans tends to contain far less saturated fat and more linoleic acid; fat provides about 35% of the dietary energy. Vegetarians differ with regard to other aspects of lifestyle besides diet, and this may explain their lower risk of CHD.

Moderate fish consumption has recently emerged as being negatively associated with risk of CHD in Holland [40] and the United States [41] but not in Hawaii [42] or Norway [43]. The association of eicosapentaenoic acid in platelets with decreased risk of CHD would also support the proposition that fish protects against CHD, as fish is the main dietary source of this fatty acid.

Plasma Lipoproteins: Metabolism and Dietary Intake

Plasma lipoproteins are lipid–protein complexes of density <1.21 g/ml, present in normal or abnormal plasma. They are classified in terms of their hydrated density, as determined in the preparative ultracentrifuge. Four classes of lipoprotein particles are present in the plasma of normal fasting human subjects: very low density lipoprotein (VLDL), density (d) <1.006 g/ml; intermediate density lipoprotein (IDL), d 1.006–1.019 g/ml; low density lipoprotein (LDL), d 1.019–1.063 g/ml; and high density lipoprotein (HDL), d 1.063–1.21 g/ml. Particles of a fifth class, the chylomicrons (d <1.006 g/ml), appear in the plasma a few hours after a fatty meal and are gradually cleared from the circulation.

VLDL is secreted mainly by the liver and is responsible for the endogenous transport of triglycerides to peripheral tissues (Fig. 6.3). The hepatic VLDL particle contains apolipoprotein B100 (apoB-100) and a triglyceride-rich core. As soon as nascent VLDL enters the plasma it acquires apolipoprotein C (apoC) and cholesterol ester, probably from HDL. In the capillaries of adipose tissue and muscle, the VLDL triglycerides are hydrolysed by endothelial lipoprotein lipase which is activated by apoC, resulting in 80%–90% loss of triglyceride and the loss of apoC. The product of this conversion, IDL, is relatively enriched in cholesteryl ester and contains apoB-100 and apolipoprotein E (apoE). IDL particles containing apoE are rapidly cleared from the plasma by hepatic uptake facilitated by receptors to apoE. IDL that escapes

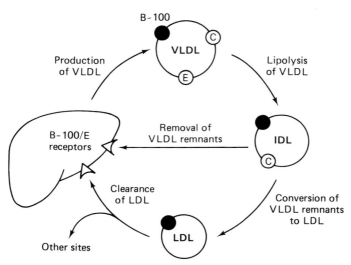

Fig. 6.3. Metabolic pathways of lipoproteins containing apoB-100. The liver produces VLDL which in circulation contains apoB-100, apoCs and apoE. VLDL triglycerides undergo lipolysis by lipoprotein lipase (LPL), and the resultant VLDL remnants, or intermediate density lipoproteins (IDL), can have two fates. They can be cleared via LDL receptors (B-100/E receptors), or they can be converted to LDL. LDL also is removed by the same receptors. Most LDL is cleared by the liver, but small quantities are cleared by extrahepatic tissue. (From [44].)

hepatic uptake and is further delipidated loses its apoE to form LDL [44]. The LDL particle is enriched in cholesterol ester and contains apoB-100. Although there is a product–precursor relationship between VLDL and LDL, not all VLDL is destined to form LDL; it appears that only the smaller size VLDL particles skip through to form LDL [45].

The concentration of LDL in plasma is dependent not only on its rate of formation but on its rate of removal. Two thirds of the LDL particles are metabolised after binding to a specific receptor for apoB-100 located on the surface of liver cells and other body cells [46]. Binding leads to cellular uptake and lysosomal degradation of the LDL by receptor-mediated endocytosis. This receptor-mediated uptake process satisfies the cholesterol needs of the cells, and keeps cholesterol synthesis suppressed by inhibiting the activity of HMGCoA reductase, the rate-limiting enzyme involved in the formation of cholesterol. In normal human subjects the remaining third of the LDL that is not taken up by the receptors is metabolised by alternative receptor-independent mechanisms. It is uptake by receptor-independent mechanisms that is associated with foam cell formation and atherosclerosis.

The rates of synthesis and removal of LDL and the VLDL–IDL–LDL cascade have been studied using radioactively labelled autologous lipoproteins. These studies show that the fractional catabolic rate (FCR) of LDL decreases with age, and that this probably accounts for the increase in LDL concentration with age [47]. Dietary factors that increase the synthesis of VLDL do not necessarily increase LDL concentrations. For example, a high sugar intake decreases the proportion of VLDL converted into LDL [48]. Nor are reductions in VLDL synthesis necessarily accompanied by a fall in LDL concentrations. For example, in patients with type V hyperlipidaemia, where there is excessive production of VLDL, LDL concentrations tend to be low, but when VLDL synthesis is reduced either by dietary means or by drugs then LDL concentrations rise [49].

The transport of exogenous lipid differs from the endogenous pathway. Dietary fatty acids (>C10), together with dietary cholesterol, are incorporated as triglycerides into chylomicrons in the small intestine. Chylomicrons are similar to VLDL except that they contain apoB-48 instead of apoB-100. They acquire apoE and apoC from HDL in circulation. The triglycerides are hydrolysed by endothelial lipoprotein lipase leaving a chylomicron remnant. The chylomicron remnant is rapidly cleared by uptake into the liver through receptor-mediated endocytosis, which recognises its apoE. Chylomicron remnant particles are not converted to LDL. A high intake of dietary fat can compromise the endogenous lipoprotein pathway by competitively inhibiting the clearance and uptake of lipoproteins.

HDL plays a central role in plasma lipid transport, providing a reservoir of apoC and acting as a scavenger of surplus cholesterol and phospholipids.

As most of the cholesterol is carried by LDL, an elevation of plasma cholesterol usually signifies an elevation of LDL. However, in heavy drinkers elevation of plasma cholesterol may be associated with an increase in the HDL fraction. Familial hypercholesterolaemia is associated with a greatly increased risk of CHD. In these patients, LDL levels are elevated owing to an inherited defect in the receptor-mediated clearance mechanism coupled with a high synthetic rate of LDL. Atherosclerosis is present from an early age, but it differs morphologically from that seen in the general population. Elevations of certain other plasma lipoproteins, notably VLDL and IDL, are also associated with increased risk of CHD. Elevations of VLDL and IDL are associated with elevated plasma triglyceride concentrations. Low levels of HDL cholesterol often accompany high levels of VLDL and non-insulin-dependent diabetes.

Most investigators believe that chylomicrons are not atherogenic. These lipoproteins contain mainly triglycerides and little cholesterol. Moreover, familial hyperchylomicronaemia is not associated with an increased risk of atherosclerosis.

It is difficult to explain why LDL, IDL and VLDL are atherogenic. There is some evidence that VLDL is toxic to the vascular endothelium [50]. In the presence of high concentrations of lipoproteins, macrophages become engorged with lipid. These macrophages may then become trapped inside the vascular endothelium and generate chemotactic substances that attract other white cells and platelets and lead to smooth muscle cell proliferation.

The plasma lipoprotein environment seems to influence platelet reactivity. Platelet malondialdehyde formation, which is primarily an indicator of prostaglandin synthesis, is higher in hyperlipidaemic patients (Frederickson types IIA, IIb, IV) than in healthy controls [51]. However, platelet thromboxane B_2 production is enhanced by type II hyperlipidaemia but not by type IV hyperlipidaemia [52]. Although individual lipoprotein fractions have been blamed, it is important to remember that levels of several other plasma factors known to increase platelet reactivity are higher in patients with hyperlipidaemia. For example fibrinogen and clotting factors VII and VIII are increased in hypertriglyceridaemia and are lowered on treatment of the hypertriglyceridaemia with a fat-modified diet [53]. Platelets from patients with either type IV or type IIA or IIB hyperlipidaemia are less sensitive to the inhibitory effects of prostacyclin [54]. These observations imply that hyperlipidaemia increases the susceptibility of the blood vessel wall to damage by thrombotic events.

Quantifying the Influence of Fat on Plasma Lipoprotein Concentrations

The major argument for indicting saturated fat intake in the causation of CHD is that variations in median plasma cholesterol concentrations between countries can largely be explained by differences in saturated fat intake. For example, in the Seven Countries Study, 59% of the variation in the median serum cholesterol concentration between countries could be explained by differences in the intakes of saturated fatty acids and cholesterol. In contrast to this, most intrapopulation studies suggest that differences in dietary fat intake explain only a small part of the variability in plasma cholesterol in the population [15,55]

Cholesterol in the diet has a trivial effect on plasma cholesterol concentrations. The first 200 mg are the most effective in raising plasma cholesterol levels [56]. Over the range of practical intake (0–400 mg cholesterol/day), each 100 mg of cholesterol in the diet leads to an increase in plasma cholesterol of about 4 mg/100 ml [57]. High dietary intakes of cholesterol are believed to decrease the number of LDL receptors in the liver and thus reduce the fractional catabolic rate of LDL [58].

In the 1950s and 1960s Keys carried out a series of studies on the effects of different types of fat on total cholesterol in healthy volunteers. He noted that saturated fatty acids, 12–16 carbon atoms long, increased plasma cholesterol, and that polyunsaturated fatty acids (linoleic acid) lowered it but were only half as potent as saturated fats. Mono-unsaturated fats, as found in olive oil, had a neutral effect, neither increasing nor decreasing plasma cholesterol. These studies were carried out in healthy young volunteers using diets in which 40% of energy was derived from fat [59]. For every 1% of the energy intake as saturated fatty acid replaced by linoleic acid there is a reduction in plasma cholesterol of about 5 mg/100 ml.

Keys developed the following equation to predict changes in plasma cholesterol that occur with alterations in the dietary intake of saturated and polyunsaturated fat (all *cis*-linoleic and linolenic acids):

Change in plasma cholesterol mg/dl=1.3(2DS-DP) + SQRT(DC)

where: DS= difference in percentage energy derived from saturated fat,
DP= difference in percentage energy derived from polyunsaturated fat, and
DC=dietary cholesterol in mg/1000 kcal.

More recently studies have reinvestigated the effects of saturated, polyunsaturated and mono-unsaturated fats in patients who have suffered a heart attack, and have looked at the distribution of cholesterol in the different lipoprotein fractions [60]. The saturated fat diet (palm oil) increased total and LDL cholesterol concentrations. The polyunsaturated fat diet (safflower oil rich in linoleic acid) lowered total, LDL and HDL cholesterol concentrations. The mono-unsaturated fat diet (mutant safflower oil rich in oleic acid) lowered total cholesterol concentrations and lowered LDL cholesterol concentrations as much as the polyunsaturated fat, without lowering HDL cholesterol concentrations. The results of this study imply that it is better to replace saturated fats by mono-unsaturated rather than polyunsaturated vegetable oils.

Saturated fatty acids are believed to increase the rate of LDL synthesis, and linoleic acid was claimed to increase the fractional catabolic rate of LDL slightly in normal subjects, but not in patients with hypercholesterolaemia [61,62]. Cortese [63] argues that high intakes of linoleic acid decrease the rate of synthesis of LDL. The major effect of increasing the ratio of linoleic acid to saturated fatty acids is to decrease the rate of synthesis of LDL.

Marine oils provide a different type of polyunsaturated fatty acid to those found in vegetable oils: eicosapentaenoic acid (20:5n3; EPA) and docosahexaenoic acid (22:6n−3; DHA) are the major polyunsaturates in fish oil, whereas linoleic (18:2n−6) and linolenic (18:3n−3) acids are the major types in vegetable oils. These marine polyunsaturated fatty acids lower plasma triglyceride and cholesterol concentrations but mainly in the VLDL fraction [64].

Greenland Eskimos living on their traditional seafood diet, which provides about 5 g EPA/day and 7 g DHA/day, have moderately low levels of LDL cholesterol, very low levels of VLDL triglycerides and high levels of HDL cholesterol compared with Eskimos living on a Western diet [25]. The consumption of an Eskimo diet, mackerel (200 g/day) but not salmon, or fish oil supplements (20 g/day), increases HDL cholesterol concentrations slightly. Similar intakes markedly lower plasma triglyceride concentrations in both normal and hypertriglyceridaemic subjects, by reducing the synthesis of both triglyceride and apoB in VLDL [27]. In vitro studies have shown that EPA and DHA are reversible inhibitors of hepatic triglyceride synthesis.

Total plasma cholesterol concentrations are reduced by fish consumption, but most of the reduction occurs in the VLDL fraction. Very high intakes of fish oil (90–120 g/day) do lower the concentration of both LDL cholesterol and LDL apoB by decreasing the rate of LDL synthesis. Such high intakes also prevent the rise in plasma cholesterol obtained with dietary cholesterol. However, at lower intakes (15 g/day) there is a tendency for LDL cholesterol and LDL apoB concentration to rise, particularly in patients with type V hyperlipoproteinaemia [65,66]. A likely explanation is that a moderate intake of fish oil decreases hepatic triglyceride synthesis, so that smaller than normal VLDL particles are secreted. These small particles are known to be more readily converted to LDL than the larger triglyceride-rich ones. On the one hand, the reduction in VLDL synthesis with fish diets is probably beneficial with regard to risk of atherosclerosis, whereas the increase in LDL concentration might be regarded as deleterious.

Trans isomers are formed during the industrial and biological hydrogenation of unsaturated fats. Margarines and other processed fats can contain relatively high proportions of these isomers. Dairy fat and the fat from lamb and beef also contain *trans* isomers. A number of studies have evaluated the influence of *trans* fatty acids on plasma cholesterol concentrations in man. The majority of these have used industrially hardened vegetable oils. Only one study has employed partially hydrogenated marine oils.

A preliminary communication by Vergroesen in 1972 [67] is often quoted as showing that elaidic acid (18:1 *trans*) increases plasma cholesterol concentrations relative to oleic acid (18:1 *cis*). It was thought that elaidic acid had an intermediate effect on plasma cholesterol between that of *cis* mono-unsaturated fatty acids and saturated fatty acids. Two studies were carried out using liquid formula diets providing 13% of energy as elaidic acid. In the control diet, the elaidic acid was replaced by oleic acid. The first study investigated the effect of elaidic acid with and without additional dietary cholesterol on plasma cholesterol concentration. The authors admit [68] the study was not "flawless" because serum cholesterol concentrations fluctuated markedly in an untreated control group. Moreover, the results of the study did not achieve statistical significance at the 5% level. This first study showed that elaidic acid did not increase plasma cholesterol, except in the presence of dietary cholesterol. However, in the second study, elaidic acid given with dietary cholesterol had the same effect on plasma cholesterol as the control diet. The latter finding is in agreement with the more recent studies. The following conclusions can be drawn : saturated fatty acids have a greater cholesterol-raising effect than do *trans* fatty acids; *trans* polyunsaturated fatty acids do not lower the plasma cholesterol concentration in the way all-*cis* polyunsaturated fatty acids do; *trans* 9–18:1 has an equivalent effect on plasma cholesterol to that of *cis* 9:1; the influence of 16:1 *trans* isomers on plasma cholesterol is unknown; *trans* fatty acids provided as partially hydrogenated vegetable oils and consumed in amounts ranging from 3% to 14% of total energy, have little influence on plasma cholesterol concentrations in man [69].

Several studies have also looked at the effect of reducing the level of total fat in the diet to between 25% and 30% of the energy intake. Again it appears that the key factor in lowering plasma cholesterol is a reduction in the intake of saturated fat. Increasing the proportion of linoleic acid from 4% to 10% of total energy had little additional benefit [70].

Does Cholesterol Reduction Decrease the Risk of CHD?

Dietary treatment of hypercholesterolaemia by a combination of a modified fat intake and drug treatment does bring about a slight reduction in CHD risk. Evidence for this is derived from two major drug trials: the World Health Organisation clofibrate trial [71] and the Lipid Research Clinics cholestyramine trial [72]. These studies showed that benefit in terms of decreased risk of CHD applied to individuals in the top quintile; subjects with moderate elevation of plasma cholesterol showed no benefit. It was estimated that for each 1 mg/100 ml that cholesterol was reduced there was a 2% reduction in risk from CHD. The conclusions from these studies on subjects with hypercholesterolaemia have dubiously been extrapolated to the general population. Cholesterol reduction by pharmacological means is not without side effects. In the clofibrate trial there was an increased incidence of liver and biliary disease. Moreoever, there was an excess total mortality in the drug-treated group. While there is evidence that lipid-lowering therapy benefits patients with severe hypercholesterolaemia, it may not be appropriate to extrapolate this conclusion to what can be obtained by dietary means in the general population.

Dietary Fat and Thrombotic Tendency

Dietary fat intake may affect the development of atherosclerosis by influencing thrombotic tendency. Alterations in thrombotic tendency may have short-term effects by influencing risk of coronary thrombosis. Post-prandial lipaemia can cause platelets to aggregate [73]. High fat intakes are also associated with an increased activity of clotting factor VII, which is a predictor of CHD [74]. Hornstra [75] has shown that most saturated fats increase thrombotic tendency in rats whereas polyunsaturated fats, whether of vegetable or marine origin, have an opposite effect. Palm oil and cocoa butter appear to be exceptions. Butter, hardened coconut oil and medium chain triglycerides were particularly prothrombotic. Mono-unsaturated fatty acids appeared to be neutral. The thrombotic potential of partially hyrogenated soyabean oil was found to be similar to a predicted value calculated on the basis of its saturated and polyunsaturated fatty acid content. Moreover, elaidic acid 18:1 *trans* was found to be no more thrombogenic than 18:1 *cis*.

Some of the effects of dietary fat on thrombotic tendency are believed to be mediated through changes in the production of eicosanoids (prostaglandins, thromboxanes, prostacyclins and leukotrienes) (Fig. 6.4). Cyclo-oxygenase metabolites of arachiodonic acid (20:4n−6; AA), with opposing effects and produced in different locations, are believed to regulate platelet behaviour at the site of injury: thromboxane A_2 produced by platelets causes platelet aggregation and vasoconstriction; prostacyclin PGI_2 produced by the vascular endothelium counteracts the effects of thromboxane A_2. Coronary atherosclerosis decreases the capacity to produce prostacyclin, so that the balance between thromboxane and prostacyclin is altered in a direction that increases the risk of coronary thrombosis [76]. This view is supported by the observation that aspirin, which inhibits cyclo-oxygenase and platelet thromboxane production, halves the risk of myocardial infarction in patients with unstable angina [77]. AA is also converted to other important metabolites by platelets and polymorph neutrophils by way of the lipoxygenase pathway, which is not inhibited by aspirin. These metabolites, particularly leukotriene B_4, are strongly chemotactic

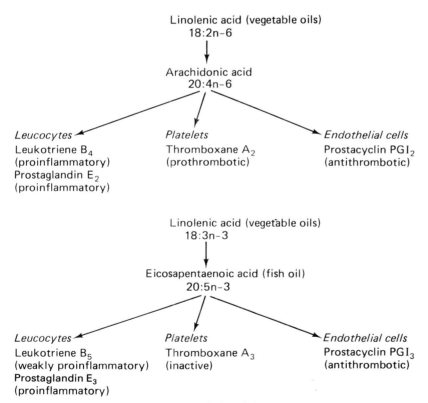

Fig. 6.4.   Eicosanoids formed from arachidonic and eicosapentaenoic acids.

to leucocytes and may be responsible for the massive leucocyte migration into the myocardium that occurs in the vicinity of an experimental coronary occlusion. The ability of EPA partially to inhibit both cyclo-oxygenase and lipoxygenase pathways may explain the decreased infarct volume observed in dogs treated with fish oils in whom myocardial infarction was experimentally induced compared with controls [78].

Eicosanoids can be formed from EPA, but they tend to be less active than those derived from AA. For example, thromboxane A_3 and leukotriene B_5 are less active than thromboxane A_2 and leukotriene B_4, but prostacyclin PGI_3 is as active as prostacyclin PGI_2. Thromboxane B_3, prostacyclin I_3 and leukotriene B_5 have been detected after feeding massive amounts of fish (400–800 g mackerel/day) or large amounts of fish oil (20–50 g/day) [79]. These observations support the hypothesis that EPA modulates the production of active eicosanoids in a way that would decrease both thrombotic and inflammatory reactions.

The effect linoleic acid has on platelet aggregation depends upon the amount consumed. A dietary deficiency of linoleic acid, i.e. less than 1% of the energy intake, decreases the amount of AA in both platelet and arterial wall lipids [75]. Subsequently the capacity to produce both thromboxane A_2 and prostacyclin PGI_2 is reduced, prostaglandin-mediated platelet aggregation does not occur and arterial thrombotic tendency is low. Dietary linoleic acid restores the level of AA in platelet and arterial lipids, prostaglandin production and platelet aggregation. Tendency to arterial thrombosis is maximised with a linoleic acid intake in the region of 6% of the energy intake. However, increasing intakes above this level leads to a reduction in thrombotic tendency. Human intakes of linoleic acid are normally in the range 4%–10% of the energy intake.

Measurements of platelet aggregation have shown that farmers with high intakes of dairy fats have a high response to thrombin compared with farmers who mainly consume vegetable oils [80]. It was possible to reduce the sensitivity of platelets to aggregating agents by decreasing the total fat intake, and partially replacing the dairy fats with vegetable oils and margarine rich in linoleic acid [81,82]. In these studies it is impossible to discriminate between the effects of a decreased saturated fat intake and those of an increased linoleic acid intake. Moreover, as edible oils were used rather than pure fatty acids, it is possible that the effects could be attributed to other constituents in the oils.

Atherosclerosis in Animals

It is possible to induce a form of atherosclerosis in animals by feeding large amounts of cholesterol in the diet, usually 1%–2% by weight of diet. This is a concentration 50–100 times greater than that in human diets. It is now accepted by most authorities that the lesions seen in such cholesterol-treated animals are unlike those seen in man. Human hypercholesterolaemia is characterised by increased concentrations of LDL, whereas cholesterol-induced hypercholesterolaemia in experimental animals is associated with the production of cholesteryl ester-rich lipoproteins ($d<1.006$) with β-electrophoretic mobility (β-VLDL) [83]. β-VLDL may represent remnants of the intestinal lipoproteins, or may be synthesised by the liver in response to the delivery of excessive amounts of cholesterol to this organ. β-VLDL will cause macrophages to accumulate massive amounts of cholesteryl esters, which resemble foam cells in the arterial wall. Rabbits, pigs and certain primates when fed diets containing a relatively high proportion of saturated fat over a long period of time, do develop lesions that are more similar to those in man. More recent models involve causing injury to the arterial endothelium coupled with diets high in fat and cholesterol.

The severity of experimental atherosclerosis is influenced by the type, rather than the quantity, of fat in the diet. When vegetable oils such as sunflower seed oil are substituted for butter fat, this is accompanied by less atherosclerosis. However, results in animals have been notoriously variable. For example, early reports suggested that peanut oil was highly atherogenic when fed to monkeys, but more recent, carefully controlled studies show it to have low atherogenic potential [84]. Generally saturated fats such as butter, tallow, lard and hardened coconut oil have been found to be atherogenic. Palm oil and cocoa butter appear to be exceptions. Mono-unsaturated fatty acids do not appear to be atherogenic in animals.

Early studies suggested that industrially hydrogenated fats were more atherogenic than beef tallow. However, the experimental diets used were deficient in linoleic acid. Later studies, which used diets that supplied an adequate intake of linoleid acid, showed there was no increase in the incidence of atherosclerosis. Kritchevsky [85] concludes that *trans* fatty acids, resulting from the industrial hydrogenation of vegetable oils, when fed in amounts up to 14% of the energy intake, are not atherogenic. This is in contrast to certain saturated fatty acids such as 14:0 which are known to be atherogenic. The influence of partially hydrogenated fish oil on atherosclerosis has been less thoroughly studied. Schiefer [86] did not find atherosclerotic lesions in primates fed partially hydrogenated fish oil. Mueller et al. [87] also comment on the low atherogenicity of hardened marine oil in primates. The observation that *trans* fatty acids are not atherogenic, like certain saturated fatty acids, even though they do raise plasma cholesterol levels in animals, may also reflect differences with regard to their effects on thrombotic tendency.

Polyunsaturated fatty acids from fish oils inhibit atherogenesis in pigs [88] and dogs [89] even in the presence of hypercholesterolaemia. It seems that fish oil offers protection against atherosclerosis by a mechanism that overrides the influence of plasma lipoproteins. For example, intimal hyperplasia of vein grafts from hypercholesterolaemic dogs is inhibited by the feeding of fish oil. Protection may be afforded by changes in eicosanoid metabolism.

Trials of Diet in the Prevention of CHD

A number of trials have been carried out to test whether changing the nature of dietary fat intake in middle life reduces the risk of death from CHD. Interpretation of these trials is fraught with problems. The dietary regimens varied, as did the age and type of patients in the trial. The statistical power of many trials was limited by sample size. Multiple risk factor intervention trials have also been undertaken, in which individuals judged as being at high risk of developing CHD (as predicted by blood pressure, serum cholesterol measurements and smoking habits), were allocated to groups receiving either special intervention or "usual care". In the MRFIT [90] study, no difference was observed in CHD mortality between the group that received special intervention and the group that were left to die in their own time. In the United

Kingdom, a similar type of study led to a high incidence of coronary death in the special intervention group compared with the control group [91]. This could perhaps be interpreted as meaning that the subjects were receiving the wrong advice.

The generally held view has been that dietary intervention in middle life has a small impact on CHD mortality and for intervention to be effective it must be started in early adult life. Nevertheless, it is worth while examining three well-controlled trials which showed benefit from changes in fat intake over a relatively short period of time. The first of these was the Oslo Heart Study [92], which was a secondary prevention trial. Subjects were allocated to control or experimental diets. The saturated fat intake was markedly restricted in this study and was partially replaced by polyunsaturated fat of both vegetable and marine origin. Total fat accounted for 39% of the energy intake, saturated fat 8.4%, linoleic acid 15.5%, linolenic acid 2.6%, and other polyunsaturated fatty acids from fish 2.4% of the energy intake. After 5 years the incidence of myocardial infarction and angina was significantly lower in the experimental group compared with the controls. Sudden cardiac death was similar between the two groups. Total CHD mortality was lower in the experimental group, but this did not achieve statistical significance. The dietary intervention showed no benefit in subjects over the age of 60 years. Benefit in terms of reduced incidence of angina and myocardial infarction was evident in those non-smoking subjects without hypertension in whom cholesterol was initially elevated. Plasma cholesterol levels were reduced from a mean of 296 mg/100 ml to 244 mg/100 ml.

As a follow-up to this trial, a primary prevention trial was undertaken in younger men with high plasma cholesterol concentrations. Dietary advice was given and the subjects were urged to give up smoking [93]. Total fat intake was reduced from 44% to 28% of the dietary energy and saturated fatty acid intakes were reduced from 18% to 8% of the dietary energy. Serum cholesterol fell from a mean of 329 to 286 mg/100ml and the rate of fatal and non-fatal infarctions was reduced by nearly half. The reduction in CHD risk was greater than could be predicted from giving up smoking alone, and the reduction in risk was proportional to the reduction in plasma cholesterol concentration. Total mortality was not statistically significantly different. However, the statistical power of the study with regard to this variable was not high for the number of subjects studied.

A cross-over design trial of two diets, both providing 40% energy from fat, was carried out in two mental hospitals in Finland [94]. In this study polyunsaturated fats, mainly soya bean oil and sunflower oil margarine, replaced butter and animal fats in the diet. This change was accompanied by a reduction in death from CHD, and there was evidence of reduced sensitivity of platelets to aggregation. Total mortality in this trial was unaffected.

The studies imply that risk of death from CHD can be reduced by short-term intervention. However, there was a trend for non-cardiovascular mortality rates to increase in some trials where linoleic acid replaced saturated fats in the diet so that the intake of linoleic acid was increased to about 16% of the energy intake.

Conclusions

Current dietary advice given by the British Department of Health and Social Security (DHSS), for the general population, recommends maintenance of ideal body weight, a reduction in total fat intake to 35% of energy intake, and a reduction in saturated fat intake from 20% to 15% of energy intake, with a long-term goal of 10%. The DHSS report suggested that *trans* fatty acids should be regarded as equivalent to saturated fatty acids with respect to recommendations made for the prevention of heart disease, but failed to explain the reasoning behind this recommendation. Although there are similarities between the metabolism of *trans* fatty acids and that of saturated fatty acids, they differ with respect to their atherogenic and thrombogenic potential. Consequently, there is no good scientific basis for including *trans* fatty acids with saturated fatty acids as regards recommendations for the prevention of CHD.

Most of the saturated fat in the British diet is derived from milk products and butter. The second largest source is fatty meat and meat products. Both milk and meat play an important role in the nutrition of Western countries. Consequently it would be unreasonable, and politically unacceptable, to expect the population to give up eating these foods. The DHSS suggests several ways of achieving its recommendations: change from full cream to semi-skimmed milk or better still to skimmed milk; substitute a margarine or a low-fat spread with a low content of saturated fatty acids for butter; use vegetable oils low in saturated fatty acids, such as sunflower or olive oil, in place of other hard fats; choose lean meat and fish.

The population approach to the prevention of CHD is attractive but it is important that it be based on sound reasoning. The changes in dietary fat recommended for the general population are extremely modest, and might at the most decrease the mean serum cholesterol concentration by 14 mg/100ml. Extrapolating from the drug trials, probably inappropriately, this would be predicted to decrease the risk of CHD by about 28%. However, there is little evidence that individuals with serum cholesterol concentrations below 200 mg/100 ml will benefit from cholesterol reduction. Benefit in terms of decreased CHD mortality is proportional to the degree of serum cholesterol reduction. The aim, therefore, should be to identify and treat those with high levels effectively. The logic that a small, uniform reduction in serum cholesterol concentration in the whole population will markedly decrease the risk of CHD is like expecting the problem of alcoholism to disappear by everyone having one less drink a week : it is the distribution that needs to be altered. The European Atherosclerosis Society [95] suggests dietary intervention in subjects with a plasma cholesterol concentration greater than 200 mg/100 ml. As the median plasma cholesterol concentration of teenagers is low, about 150 mg/100 ml, the public's concern about the level of fat in children's diets might be misplaced. The question of why plasma cholesterol concentrations rise with age has not been adequately answered. It may be related to the acquisition of a "middle-age spread". Moderately elevated plasma cholesterol concentrations can be decreased without drugs in many middle-aged subjects by decreasing the intake of saturated fatty acid and by losing excess body fat. The current evidence suggests that mono-unsaturated fats, such as olive oil, may be better substitutes for saturated fats in these patients than vegetable oils. From the foregoing it can be seen that there are major flaws in the logic behind the dietary recommendations. The dietary advice advocated for the general population may well be correct but probably for the wrong reasons. The influence of dietary fat intake on thrombotic processes may be more important than its influence on plasma cholesterol concentrations.

The hypothesis that the balance between n−3 and n−6 fatty acids may modulate susceptibility to CHD is intriguing and requires further investigation. A high intake of EPA and DHA seems a plausible explanation for the low incidence of coronary artery disease amongst the Eskimos. Their extreme dietary practices are interesting because they shed light on the mechanisms leading to coronary artery disease, but it does not follow that such diets should be advocated for the general population. Although there are reasons for believing that fish oil might be of benefit to patients with thrombogenic disorders, the necessary clinical trials have yet to be carried out.

Fish used to be an important part of the British diet. It had the advantage of being available throughout the year. For religious reasons it was eaten on Fridays and other "fish days", and during Lent almost daily. Lord Trenchard [96] in his review of consumption patterns concluded that the decrease in fish consumption was one of the major changes in the British diet this century. Cod-liver oil supplements were also widely used until the 1950s. Kromhout [40] recently claimed that eating fish once or twice weekly would reduce the risk of coronary heart disease. In this prospective study a reduction in risk was found with an average daily intake of 30 g fish (two thirds white fish, one third oily), an amount that would provide far less EPA and DHA than the minimum shown to influence either plasma lipid concentrations or eicosanoid production. Fish contains several nutrients and foreign compounds that are scarce in other foods. Consequently fish might be providing some other, yet to be identified, protective factor.

In conclusion, the relationship between fat intake and CHD is complex. The evidence suggests that it is primarily the type of fat consumed, rather than the amount, that is important in affecting both thrombotic tendency and plasma lipoprotein concentrations. The degree and geometry of unsaturation and chain length seem to influence factors associated with the development of CHD. We do not yet know why this is so.

Summary

1. The relationship between fat intake and CHD is complex because susceptibility is influenced by several other factors.

2. The evidence suggests that it is primarily the type of fat consumed rather than the amount that is important.

3. Moderately elevated plasma cholesterol concentrations, which are associated with increased risk of CHD, can be decreased in middle-aged subjects by decreasing the intake of saturated fatty acids and by losing excess body weight.

References

1. DHSS (1984) Diet and cardiovascular disease. Reports on health and social subjects 28. HMSO, London
2. Marmot MG (1979) Epidemiological basis for the prevention of coronary heart disease. Bull WHO 57:331–347
3. Thom TJ, Epstein FH, Feldman JJ, Leaverton PE (1985) Trends in total mortality and mortality from heart disease in 26 countries from 1950 to 1978. Int J Epidemiol 14:510–520

4. Kromann N, Green A (1980) Epidemiological studies in the Upernavik District, Greenland. Acta Med Scand 208:401–406
5. Marmot MG (1984) Immigrant mortality in England and Wales 1970–78. Study of medical and population subjects. 47 OPCS:HMSO, London
6. Beckles GLA, Miller GJ, Kirkwood BR et al. (1986) High total and cardiovascular disease mortality in adults of Indian descent in Trinidad, unexplained by major coronary risk factors. Lancet II:1298–1300
7. Barker DJP, Osmond C (1986) Infant mortality, childhood nutrition, and ischaemic heart disease in England and Wales. Lancet I:1077–1081
8. Marmot MG, Syme SL, Kato H, Cohen JB, Belsky J (1975) Epidemiological studies of coronary heart disease and stroke in Japanese men living in Japan, Hawaii and California. Am J Epidemiol 102:514–525
9. Medalie JH, Khan NA, Neufeld NH et al. (1983) Myocardial infarction over a five-year period. I. Prevalence, incidence and mortality experienced. J Chron Dis 26:63–84
10. Kannel WB, Gordon T (1970) Some characteristics related to incidence of cardiovascular death: Framingham study, 16-year follow-up. US Government Printing Office, Washington DC
11. Goldbourt U, Neufeld HN (1986) Genetic aspects of arteriosclerosis. Arteriosclerosis 6:357–377
12. Townsend JL, Meade TW (1979) Ischaemic heart disease mortality risks for smokers and non-smokers. J Epidemiol Community Health 33:243–247
13. Keys A (1970) Coronary heart disease in seven countries. Circulation 41:1–211
14. Pooling Project Research (1978) Relationship of blood pressure, serum cholesterol, smoking habit, relative weight and ECG abnormalities to incidence of major coronary events: final report of the Pooling Project. J Chron Dis 31:201–306
15. Cambien F, Jaqueson A, Richard JL, Warnet JM, Ducimetiere P, Claude JF (1983) Is the level of serum triglyceride a significant predictor of coronary death in normocholesterolemic subjects? Am J Epidemiol 124:624–632
16. Stern MP, Haffner SM (1986) Body fat distribution and hyperinsulinemia as risk factors for diabetes and cardiovascular disease. Arteriosclerosis 6:123–130
17. Mather HM, Keen H (1985) The Southall diabetes survey. Prevalence of known diabetes in Asians and Europeans. Br Med J 291:1081–1084
18. Miller GJ, Miller NE (1975) Plasma-high-density-lipoprotein concentration and development of ischaemic heart disease. Lancet I:16–19
19. Teng B, Thompson GR, Sniderman AD, Forter TM, Krauss RM, Kwiterovich PO (1983) Composition and distribution of low density lipoprotein fractions in hyperapobetalipoproteinemia, normolipidemia, and familial hypercholesterolemia. Proc Natl Acad Sci USA 80:6662–6666
20. Laakso M, Voutilainen E, Pyorala K, Sarlund H (1985) Association of low HDL and HDL2 cholesterol with coronary heart disease in noninsulin-dependent diabetics. Arteriosclerosis 5:653–658
21. Meade TW, Chakrabarti R, Haines AP et al. (1980) Haemostatic function and cardiovascular death: early results of a prospective study. Lancet I:1050–1054
22. Ross R, Faggiotto A, Bowen-Pope D, Raines E (1984) The role of endothelial injury and platelet and macrophage interactions in atherosclerosis. Circulation 70:77
23. Smith EB (1985) Lipoproteins and atheroma. In: Kakkar VV (ed) Atheroma and thrombosis. Academic Press, London, pp 22–25
24. Maseri A, L'Abbate A, Baroldi G et al. (1978) Coronary vasospasm as a possible cause of myocardial infarction. A conclusion derived from preinfarction angina. N Engl J Med 299:1271–1277
25. Bang HO, Dyerberg J (1980) Lipid metabolism in Greenland Eskimos. Adv Nutr Res 3:1–40
26. Prior IM, Evans JG (1970) Current developments in the Pacific. In: Jones RJ (ed) Atherosclerosis II. Proceedings of the Second International Symposium. Springer-Verlag, Berlin Heidelberg New York, pp 335–342
27. Sanders TAB (1987) Fish and coronary artery disease. Br Heart J 57:214–219
28. McGill HC (1979) The relationship of dietary cholesterol to serum cholesterol and atherosclerosis in man. Am J Clin Nutr 32:2664–2702
29. Phillips RL, Lemon FR, Beeson WL, Kuzma JW (1978) Coronary heart disease mortality among Seventh-Day Adventists with different dietary habits: a preliminary report. Am J Clin Nutr 31:191–198
30. Logan RL, Thomson MR, Riemersma RA et al. (1984) Risk factors for ischaemic heart disease in normal men aged 40. Lancet I:949–955
31. Wood DA, Riemersma RA, Butler S et al. (1987) Linoleic and eicosapentaenoic acids in adipose tissue and platelets and risk of coronary heart disease. Lancet I:117–183
32. Sanders TAB, Ellis FR, Dickerson JWT (1978) Studies of vegans: the fatty acids composition of plasma choline phosphoglycerides, erythrocytes, adipose tissue, and breast milk, and some indi-

cators of susceptibility to ischemic heart disease in vegans and omnivore controls. Am J Clin Nutr 31:805–813

33. Reddy S, Sanders TAB (1987) Plasma phospholipid fatty acid composition in men of Asian and European descent. Proc Nutr Soc 46:117 (abstract)

34. Thomas LH, Jones PR, Winter JA, Smith H (1981) Hydrogenated oils and fats: presence of chemically-modified fatty acids in human adipose tissue. Am J Clin Nutr 34:877–886

35. Burr ML, Sweetnam PM (1982) Vegetarianism, dietary fiber, and mortality. Am J Clin Nutr 36:873–877

36. Margetts BM, Beilin LJ, Vandongen R, Armstrong BK (1986) Vegetarian diet in mild hypertension: a randomised controlled trial. Br Med J 293:1468–1471

37. Haines AP, Chakrabarti R, Fisher D, Meade TW, North WRS, Stirling Y (1980) Haemostatic variables in vegetarians and non-vegetarians. Thromb Res 19:139–148

38. Burr ML, Bates CJ, Fehily AM, St Leger AS (1981) Plasma cholesterol and blood pressure in vegetarians. J Hum Nutr 35:437–441

39. Roshanai F, Sanders TAB (1984) Assessment of fatty acid intakes in vegans and omnivores. Hum Nutr Appl Nutr 38A:345–354

40. Kromhout D, Bosschieter EB, Coulander CL (1984) The inverse relation between fish consumption and 20-year mortality from coronary disease. N Engl J Med 312:1205–1209

41. Shekelle RB, Missell L, Oglesby P et al. (1985) Fish consumption and mortality from cardiovascular disease. N Engl J Med 313:820

42. Vollset SE, Heuch I, Bjelke E (1985) Fish consumption and mortality from cardiovascular disease. N Engl J Med 313:820–821

43. Curb JD, Reed DM (1985) Fish consumption and mortality from cardiovascular disease. N Engl J Med 313:821–822

44. Grundy SM (1984) Pathogenesis of hyperlipoproteinemia. J Lipid Res 25:1611–1618

45. Packard CJ, Munro A, Lorimer AR, Gotto AM, Shepherd J (1984) Metabolism of apolipoprotein B in large triglyceride-rich very low density lipoproteins of normal and hypertriglyceridemic subjects. J Clin Invest 75:2178–2192

46. Goldstein JL, Brown MS (1984) Progress in understanding the LDL receptor and HMG-CoA reductase, two membrane proteins that regulate the plasma cholesterol. J Lipid Res 25:1450–1461

47. Miller NE (1984) Why does plasma low density lipoprotein concentration in adults increase with age? Lancet I:263–266

48. Nestel PJ, Reardon M, Fidge NH (1979) Sucrose-induced changes in VLDL- and LDL-B apoprotein removal rates. Metabolism 28:531–535

49. Manzato E, Marin R, Gasparotto A et al. (1986) Lipoprotein modifications during dietary treatment in patients with primary type V hyperlipoproteinaemia. Eur J Clin Invest 16:149–156

50. Rudel LL, Parks JS, Johnson FL, Babiak J (1986) Low density lipoproteins in atherosclerosis. J Lipid Res 27:465–474

51. Gianturco SH, Eskin SG, Navarro LT, Lahart CJ, Smith LC, Gotto Am (1980) Abnormal effects of hypertriacylglycerolemic very low-density lipoproteins on 3-hydroxy-3-methylglutaryl-coA reductase activity and viability of cultured bovine aortic endothelial cells. Biochim Biophys Acta 618:143–152

52. Sanders TAB (1983) Dietary fat and platelet function. Clin Sci 65:343–450

53. Elkeles RS, Chakrabarti R, Vickers M, Stirling YB, Meade TW (1980) Effect of treatment of hyperlipidaemia on haemostatic variables. Br Med J 281:973

54. Strano A, Davi G, Averna M et al. (1982) Platelet sensitivity to prostacyclin and thromboxane production in hyperlipidemic patients. Thromb Haemost 48:18–20

55. Yano K, Reed DM, Curb JD, Hankin JH, Albers JJ (1986) Biological and dietary correlates of plasma lipids and lipoproteins among elderly Japanese men in Hawaii. Arteriosclerosis 6:422–433

56. Keys A (1984) Serum-cholesterol response to dietary cholesterol Am J Clin Nutr 40:351–359

57. Hegsted DM (1986) Serum-cholesterol response to dietary cholesterol: a re-evaluation. Am J Clin Nutr 44:299–305

58. Packard CJ, McKinney L, Carr K, Shepherd J (1983) Cholesterol feeding increases low density lipoprotein synthesis. J Clin Invest 72:45–51

59. Keys A, Parlin RW (1966) Serum-cholesterol response to changes in dietary lipids. Am J Clin Nutr 19:175–81

60. Mattson FH, Grundy SM (1985) Comparison of effects of dietary saturated, monounsaturated, and polyunsaturated fatty acids on plasma lipids and lipoproteins in man. J Lipid Res 26:194–202

61. Illingworth DR, Sundberg EE, Becker N, Connor WE, Alaupovic P (1981) Influence of saturated, monounsaturated and w6-PUFA on LDL metabolism in man. Arteriosclerosis 1:380

62. Turner JD, Ngoc-anh Le, Brown WV (1981) Effect of changing dietary fat saturation on low-density lipoprotein metabolism in man. Am J Physiol 241:E57–E63

63. Cortese C, Levy Y, Janus ED et al. (1983) Modes of action of lipid-lowering diets in man: studies of apolipoprotein B kinetics in relation to fat. Eur J Clin Invest 13:79–85
64. Harriss WS, Connor WE, McMurray MP (1983) The comparitive reductions of plasma lipids and lipoproteins by dietary polyunsaturated fats: salmon vs vegetable oil. Metabolism 32:179–184
65. Phillipson BE, Rothrock DW, Connor WE, Harris WS, Illingworth DR (1985) Reduction of plasma lipids, lipoproteins, and apoproteins by dietary fish oils in patients with hypertriglyceridemia. N Engl J Med 313:1210–1216
66. Sullivan DR, Sanders TAB, Trayner IM, Thompson GR (1986) Paradoxical elevation of LDL apoprotein B levels in hypertriglyceridaemic patients and normal subjects ingesting fish oil. Atherosclerosis 61:129–134
67. Vergroesen AJ (1972) Dietary fat and cardiovascular disease: possible modes of action of linoleic acid. Proc Nutr Soc 31:323–329
68. Vergroesen AJ, Gottenbos JJ (1975) The role of fats in human nutrition: an introduction. In: Vergroesen AJ (ed) The role of fats in human nutrition. Academic Press, New York, pp 1–32
69. British Nutrition Foundation (1979) Trans fatty acids. Report of the British Nutrition Foundation's Task Force. British Nutrition Foundation, London
70. Kuusi T, Ehnholm C, Huttunen JK et al. (1985) Concentration and composition of serum lipoproteins during a low-fat diet at two levels of polyunsaturated fat. J Lipid Res 26:360–367
71. Report of the committee of principal investigators (1984) WHO cooperative trial on primary prevention of ischaemic heart disease with clofibrate to lower serum cholesterol: final mortality follow-up. Lancet I:600–604
72. Lipid Research Clinics Program (1984) The Lipid Research Clinics coronary primary prevention trial results 1. Reduction in the incidence of coronary heart disease. 2. The relationship of reduction in incidence of coronary heart disease to cholesterol lowering. JAMA 251:351–64
73. O'Brien JR, Etherington MD, Jamieson S (1976) Effect of a diet of polyunsaturated fats on some platelet-function tests. Lancet II:995–997
74. Miller GJ, Martin JC, Webster J et al. (1986) Association between dietary fat intake and plasma factor VII coagulant activity – a predictor of cardiovascular mortality. Atherosclerosis 60:269–277
75. Hornstra G (1982) Dietary fats, prostanoids and arterial thrombosis. In: Developments in hematology and immunology vol 4. Martinus Nijhoff, London
76. Moncada S, Vane JR (1979) Arachidonic acid metabolites and the interactions between platelets and blood vessel walls. N Engl J Med 300:1142–1147
77. Cairns JA, Gent M, Singer J et al. (1985) Aspirin, sulfinpyrazone, or both in unstable angina. Results of a Canadian multicenter-trial. N Engl J Med 313:1369–1375
78. Culp BR, Lands WEM, Lucches BR, Pitt R, Romson J (1980) The effect of dietary supplementation of fish oil on experimental myocardial infarction. Prostaglandins 20:1021–1031
79. Knapp HR, Reilly AG, Allesandrini P, Fitzgerald GA (1986) In vivo indexes of platelet and vascular function during fish oil administration in patients with atherosclerosis. N Engl J Med 314:937–942
80. Renaud S, Morazain R, McGregor L, Baudier F (1979) Dietary fats and platelet functions in relation to atherosclerosis and coronary heart disease. Haemostasis 8:234–251
81. Renaud S, Godsey F, Dumont E, Thevenon C, Ortchanian E, Martin JL (1986) Influence of long-term diet modification on platelet function in Moselle farmers. Am J Clin Nutr 43:136–150
82. Hornstra G, Lewis B, Chait A et al. Influence of dietary fat on platelet function in men. Lancet I:115–1157
83. Mahley RW (1982) Atherogenic hyperlipoproteinemia. Med Clin N Am 66:375–402
84. Alderson LM, Hayes KC, Nicolosi RJ (1986) Peanut oil reduces diet-induced atherosclerosis in Cynomolgus Monkeys. Arteriosclerosis 6:465–474
85. Kritchevsky D (1983) Trans fatty acids in experimental atherosclerosis. Fed Proc 41:2813–2817
86. Schiefer HB (1982) Studies in non-hominid primates. In: Barlow SM, Stansby ME (eds) Nutritional evaluation of long-chain fatty acids in fish oil. Academic Press, London, pp 215–243
87. Mueller RW, Schiefer HB, Laxdal VA, Ackman RG (1982) Aortic changes in Cynomolgus monkeys fed high-fat diets (long-term study). Artery 11:174–191
88. Weiner BH, Ockene IS, Levine PH et al. (1986) Inhibition of atherosclerosis by cod-liver oil in a hyperlipidemic swine model. N Engl J Med 315:841–846
89. Landymore RW, Kinley CE, Cooper JH et al. (1985) Cod-liver oil in the prevention of intimal hyperplasia in autologous vein grafts used for arterial bypass. J Thorac Cardiovasc Surg 89:351–357
90. Multiple Risk Factor Intervention Trial Research Group (1982) Multiple risk factor intervention trial. Risk factor changes and mortality results. JAMA 248:1465–1477
91. Mitchell JRA (1985) Diet and arterial disease – the myths and realities. Proc Nutr Soc 44:363–370
92. Leren P (1966) The effect of plasma cholesterol lowering diet in male survivors of myocardial infarction. Universitetsforlaget, Oslo

93.   Hjermann I, Holme I, Byre KV, Leren P (1981) Effect of diet and smoking on the incidence of coro-
       nary heart disease. Lancet II:1301–1310
94.   Miettenen M, Turpeinen O, Karvonen MJ, Elosuo R, Paavilainen E (1972) Effect of cholesterol
       lowering diet on mortality from coronary heart disease and other causes. Lancet II:835–838
95.   European Atherosclerosis Society (1987) Stategies for the prevention of coronary heart disease: a
       policy statement of the European Atherosclerosis Society. Eur Heart J 8:77–88
96.   Lord Trenchard (1978) The interrelationship of marketing and nutrition. In: Yudkin J (ed) Diet of
       man: needs and wants. Applied Science Publishers, London, pp 225–242

Commentary

Southgate: In the discussion of risk factors there is a switch from predictors of CHD deaths to atherosclerosis. Is atherosclerosis a good predictor of CHD deaths? The relation between diet and development of atherosclerosis may be much more significant but some integration of diet over a period is required. The difficulties in assessing fat intake may be very significant in testing associations, and this section could perhaps mention the fact that food composition tables are relatively poor predictors of actual (analysed) fat intake. In particular large variations in lean to fat ratios in meat are also seen, together with large variations in individual preferences for fat consumption.

Regarding the current dietary advice given by the DHSS, surely the 35% fat target will result in variable alterations in risk, depending on level of fat intake before introducing changes? There may be two independent effects of dietary fat (or more probably overall dietary consumption): one, a long-term relationship between diet and atherosclerosis and reductions in the luminal diameter of the coronary vessels, and the other a short-term mechanism acting on platelet stickiness/thrombosis. This latter term would probably be an interaction between short-term intake of long chain polyunsaturated fatty acids and hormonal status. Since a thrombotic incident is a catastrophic (in a mathematical sense) event, it is probable that the incident is multifactorial and one in which diet at the time of the incident is a minor factor.

Jarrett: The comment in the introduction about the menopause is somewhat misleading. As Sanders' reference 3 makes clear, there is a male excess *at all ages*. The relevance of the menopause is disputed. Reference 3 is also worth more extensive quotation in the section on epidemiology. Thus in the 26 country comparison, ischaemic heart disease (IHD) mortality rates in women fell in most of the countries, or remained stable. During the period reviewed (1950–78) the sex ratio (M : F) increased in all but one country and also tended to be higher in those countries with high IHD mortality rates. Furthermore, reference 3 also points out that in women IHD mortality rates and total mortality declined by a similar degree in most countries, whereas in men IHD mortality did not follow total mortality according to any clearly discernible pattern. Thus France and England/Wales both had relatively high total mortality rates but low and high, respectively, IHD rates. This makes the comment about "Western lifestyle" too facile.

While it is true that the increased risk of CHD in Indian men in the West Indies (Sanders' reference 6) is not explained in statistical terms by traditional (*sic*) risk factors, their cholesterol levels were not low by comparison with, say, the mainland Japanese. In the Seven Countries Study, statistical predictions based on the US sample could not be applied to other populations [1]. This may be due to different genetic risks or to unknown effects of other environmental factors. *Duration* of risk factors is also an unknown quantity in prospective studies.

Sanders dismisses obesity as a risk factor, and I would agree with him, though others would not [2]. He is more sanguine about the waist/hip ratio, but quotes a prevalence study when there are two prospective studies [3,4]. One of these showed the highest risk of IHD to be in men with low Body Mass Index and high waist/hip ratio [4]! As for what he calls non-insulin-dependent diabetes I have argued that it is not a causal factor but is associated with an increased CHD risk in some undetermined fashion [5]. I await, but do not expect, refutation.

There are at least three prospective studies which have reported a positive association between measures of saturated fat intake and coronary heart disease risk [6–8] and one which reported an inverse association between the ratio of polyunsaturated to saturated fatty acids and CHD [9]. Interpretation of these findings is, of course, not straightforward, given the co-variance of the dietary constituents.

References

1. Keys A (1970) Coronary heart disease in seven countries. Circulation 41:1–211
2. Health implications of obesity: National Institutes of Health consensus development statement (1985) Ann Intern Med 103:147–151
3. Lapidus L, Bengtsson C, Larsson B et al. (1984) Distribution of adipose tissue and risk of cardiovascular disease and death: a 12 year follow-up of the participants in the population study of women in Gothenburg, Sweden. Br Med J 289:1257–1261
4. Larsson B, Svärdsudd K, Welin L et al. (1984) Abdominal adipose tissue distribution, obesity and risk of cardiovascular disease and death: a 13 year follow-up of participants in the study of men born in 1913. Br Med J 288:1401–1404
5. Jarrett RJ (1984) Type 2 (non-insulin-dependent) diabetes mellitus and coronary heart disease – chicken, egg or neither? Diabetologia 26:99–102
6. Kushi H, Lew RA, Stare FJ et al. (1985) Diet and 20-year mortality from coronary heart disease: the Ireland-Boston diet – heart study. N Engl J Med 312:811–818
7. Garcia-Palmieri MR, Sorlie P, Tillotson J et al. (1980) Relationship of dietary intake to subsequent coronary heart disease incidence; the Puerto Rico heart health program. Am J Clin Nutr 33:1818–1827
8. McGee DL, Reed DM, Yano K et al. (1984) Ten year incidence of coronary heart disease in the Honolulu heart program: relationship to nutrient intake. Am J Epidemiol 119:667–676
9. Morris JN, Marr JW, Clayton DG (1977) Diet and heart: a postscript. Br Med J ii:1307–1314

Chapter 7

Dietary Fibre and the Diseases of Affluence

D. A. T. Southgate

Introduction

Although the traditional "balanced" diet has always included some "roughage" to prevent constipation [1] the widespread acceptance of the need to include a recommendation for dietary fibre to protect against a range of diseases prevalent in Western developed countries is a relatively recent phenomenon [2,3] which can be said to date from the early seventies with the paper of Painter and Burkitt [4]. However, the concept of a protective effect of the plant cell wall constituents in the diet, "dietary fibre", probably dates from Hipsley [5].

I will discuss here the evidence for a relation between the intake of dietary fibre and the incidence of the diseases of affluence and therefore, by inference, the need to include dietary fibre in the specification for a balanced diet.

First, I will define the term "dietary fibre". The original use of the term [5] was for the major constituents of the plant cell wall – hemicelluloses, celluloses and lignin – but the definition of Trowell et al. [6,7] provides a reasonable working definition: "the sum of lignin and the (plant) polysaccharides which are not digested by the endogenous secretion of the human gastro-intestinal tract". This physiological and philosophical definition is difficult to translate into precise terms suitable for analytical measurement, but the measurement of the non-starch polysaccharides provides the closest analytical index [8]. Lignin is an important modifier of the properties of the polysaccharides but is best considered and measured separately [9]. It should be recognised that the accurate measurement of lignin in human foods is a matter of considerable difficulty [10]. Later in the discussion on the basis for the quantitative provision of dietary fibre, I will use some data derived from the use of the Southgate method for unavailable carbohydrate [11,12], values which include lignin and enzymatically resistant starch.

Hipsley [5] presents some epidemiological evidence for a protective effect of dietary fibre against toxaemia of pregnancy, but it was Painter and Burkitt [4] who first suggested that a specific pathological condition, diverticular disease, was a deficiency disease of Western society due to a low intake of dietary fibre. As the dietary fibre hypothesis developed, a wide range of diseases were claimed to be associated with a low intake and to be prevented by a high intake of dietary fibre [17]. These included obesity, cardiovascular disease, diabetes, gallstones, diverticular disease and related "pressure diseases", and large bowel cancer. The diseases tend to have a higher incidence in developed countries and a low incidence in the less affluent, developing world. Analysis of incidence within the developed countries shows that the distribution of the incidence is skewed, often towards the lower socioeconomic groups. Thus the diseases are not strictly related to affluence [14].

Perisse et al.'s [15] classical analysis of dietary composition and the gross national product shows clear evidence of dietary compositional differences related to income. Furthermore sequential analyses of dietary trends show that the type of carbohydrate consumed is closely related to economic development, so that intake of sugars, which in the Food and Agriculture Organisation classification include sucrose, glucose syrup and honeys, rises to an upper plateau with income and while that of starch falls to a trough [16].

Diets consumed in the affluent countries can be defined by three dimensions: proportion of non-protein energy intake from fat, proportion of vegetable protein in total protein, and proportion of total carbohydrate as starch [17] (Fig. 7.1). Dietary fibre content is probably closely related to proportion of total energy as starch. It is indeed possible, as suggested by Wahlquist [18], that dietary fibre content is merely a marker for a diet associated with low incidence of certain diseases.

The evidence of an association between low disease incidence and high dietary fibre intake is not proof of the dietary fibre hypothesis [19] although a high incidence and high intake would refute the hypothesis.

In the discussion of the relation of disease to dietary fibre intake that follows, it is therefore necessary to consider both the epidemiological evidence for an association between disease incidence and intake and a mechanism that links the aetiology with dietary fibre. The thesis that will be examined is that for a number of disease states there is a relation between dietary fibre intake and the incidence of the disease, and that therefore the prescription for the optimal "balanced" diet will include a specification for dietary fibre.

Mode of Action of Dietary Fibre

Heterogeneity of Dietary Fibre

Dietary fibre is not an entity with a defined composition and defined physical properties. It is a mixture of a range of complex polysaccharides organised, for the most part, into supermolecular structures in the plant cell wall and present in foods in the mixture of cell wall types found in the range of plant foods that make up the diet [20,21] (Table 7.1). The dietary fibre intake will therefore differ in composition depending on the types of foods in the actual diet. In the diets eaten in the developing countries plant cell walls provide virtually all the dietary fibre in the diet. In the British diet and that of most of the developed countries a small but significant part of the intake is derived from plant polysaccharides used as food additives. Some of these are present in their native but extracted form, others have been modified to alter their physical properties. Associated with the polysaccharides are a range of other substances: proteins, inorganic salts, and non-carbohydrate materials such as lignins,

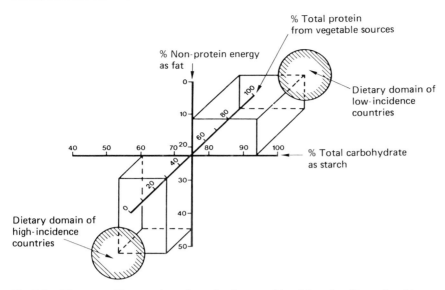

Fig. 7.1. Diagram to illustrate three-dimensional compositional domains. (Reproduced by permission of *American Journal of Clinical Nutrition*.)

Table 7.1. Principal causes of heterogeneity of dietary fibre intake

Major variable	Examples	Effects of dietary fibre
Proportions of plant food sources consumed	Cereals Vegetables Fruits	Determine types of polysaccharide present in the diet
Preparation and processing	Grinding Sieving Heat treatment (wet and dry)	Physical properties of ingested dietary fibre Physical structure of foods
Types of plant organ consumed	Roots/tubers Stems Petioles Leaves Flowers/flower buds Seeds	Types of polysaccharide present Organisation within cell wall architecture

Types of plant cell wall structures consumed	Parenchyma
	Conducting tissues:
	  phloem
	  xylem
	Supporting tissues:
	  collenchyma
	  sclerenchyma
	Epidermal tissues
		Presence of associated proteins, lignins, cutins, suberins and inorganic materials

cutins and suberins [22]. These latter substances create hydrophobic domains within and on the surfaces of the cell wall structures.

The chemistry of the major classes of compounds present in the plant cell wall has been reviewed on many occasions [20,21,25] and it is only necessary to summarise it here (Table 7.2).

Table 7.2. Source, chemistry and distribution of the components of dietary fibre

Primary source	Major groups	Components present	Summary of structures	Distribution in foods
Structural materials of the plant cell wall	Cellulose		Long chain B-glucans	All cell walls
	Non-cellulosic polysaccharides	Pectic substances	Galacturonans Arabinogalactans	Mainly in fruits and vegetables
			Arabinoxylans	Cereals
		Hemicelluloses	Glucurono-arabinoxylans	Cereals
			Glucurono-xylans	Fruits/vegetables
			Xylo-glucans	Fruits/vegetables
			B-glucans	Cereals
Non-structural polysaccharides	Gums Mucilages		Wide range of hetero polysaccharides	Seeds and Fruits
Polysaccharide food additives	Gums	Guar Locust bean	Galactomannans	Widely used in specific processed products, usually at levels below 1% by weight
	Algal polysaccharides	Alginates Carageenan	Guluro-mannuronans Sulphated-galactans	
	Modified celluloses		Carboxymethyl-1-cellulose Methylcellulose	
	Modified starches	Cross-linked Esterified		
Associated substances	Lignin		Phenypropane polymers	Most foods; increase with maturity
	Cutin Suberin		Ester of long chain hydroxy fatty acids	leaves, roots, tubers, some fruits

Dietary fibre is found in all plant foods but the ratio of dietary fibre to total metabolisable energy is extremely variable, so that the construction of a diet rich in dietary fibre has a number of constraints once one moves from diets of a semi-synthetic or experimental nature to those made up of real foods (Table 7.3). A high dietary fibre diet, in order to provide adequate energy, must include significant quantities of high extraction cereal foods and these bring with them high starch contents. High fibre diets made up solely of vegetables or fruit are extremely bulky because of the

Table 7.3. Characteristics of some typical foods providing dietary fibre

		Dietary fibre[a]		Weight of food (g) to provide 10 g DF[b]	Other constituents with 10 g DF		
		g/100 g	g/100 kcal		Fat (g)	Sugars (g)	Starch (g)
Beans	haricot, boiled	7.4	8.0	135	0.7	Trace	21.3
Cabbage	winter, boiled	2.8	18.7	360	Trace	7.9	Trace
Carrots	young, boiled	3.0	15.0	333	Trace	14.7	Trace
Potatoes	old, boiled	1.0	1.3	1000	1.0	4.0	193.0
Apples	flesh, raw	2.0	4.3	500	Trace	59.0	Trace
Plums	flesh, raw	2.9	8.1	345	Trace	40.0	Trace
Bread	white	2.7	1.2	370	6.3	6.7	6.7
Bread	wholemeal	8.5	3.9	118	3.2	2.5	2.5
Breakfast cereal	wholemeal	12.3	3.8	81	2.4	0.3	54.7
Biscuits	plain digestive	5.5	1.2	182	37.3	29.8	90.3
	chocolate-coated	3.5	0.7	285	68.7	81.2	108.3
	semi-sweet	2.3	0.5	435	106.9	97.0	228.4

[a]Values for dietary fibre include restistant starch and lignin.
[b]Dietary fibre.

Table 7.4.   Characteristics of high fibre diets

Characteristic	Comments
Bulky	Lower physical density (g/ml)
Energy density	Lower metabolisable energy per unit weight (kcal/kg), but only when fat intakes are also lower
Starch	Ratio of complex carbohydrates to simple sugars increased
Lower fat	In the context of diets over the world as a whole, the fat also tends to be primarily from vegetable sources and more polyunsaturated
Protein	Vegetable protein sources are more important than animal ones

high water content. All non-manufactured high fibre foods are low in fat. Thus we have a number of characteristics of a high fibre diet that are not totally independent of dietary fibre [17] (Table 7.4).

Physiological Effects

Dietary fibre acts at all levels in the gastrointestinal tract and effects at several levels have definite or plausible links with the aetiology of the diseases that are our concern (Fig. 7.2).

Effects on Ingestion

High fibre diets have a general property of having both a lower energy density (kcal/kg diet) and a lower physical density (kg/litre) and thus at isocaloric intakes a high fibre diet will demand the ingestion of a greater weight and volume of food [23]. Gastric capacity may be limiting in relation to energy needs, particularly in children. This is only true for diets composed of traditional foods in which low fat content is also a characteristic of such a high fibre diet. The physical structure of a diet containing plant foods is such that it has to be masticated in order to reduce it to particles of a size that can be swallowed. The times for consumption therefore tend to be longer compared with those of a diet of intrinsically lower particle size.

Gastric Effects

The bulky high fibre diet, together with the associated starch, hydrates when mixed with the gastric secretions, increasing gastric bulk. Viscous gel-forming polysaccharides of the guar gum type consumed in a dry or partially hydrated form will fully hydrate in the stomach and when fed at high levels to animals can form large boluses of material that remain in the stomach and can disturb water and electrolyte status. Gastric emptying of the less soluble components of the diet tends to be slower than that of soluble material, and studies with rats on high insoluble fibre intakes show a progressive increase in fibre content of the gastric contents after meal feeding [24]. Studies in man have not demonstrated unequivocally an effect of dietary fibre on

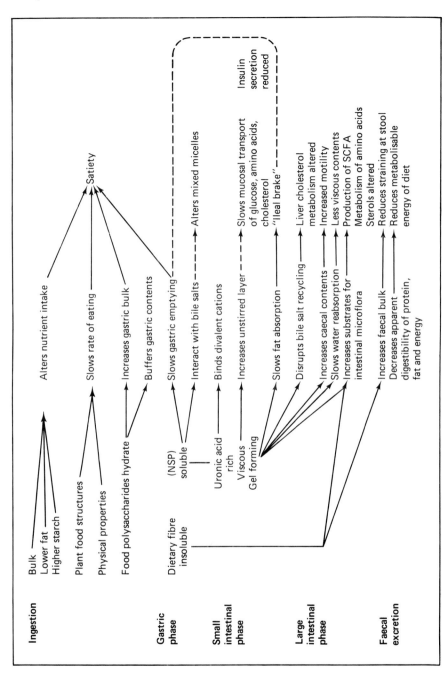

Fig. 7.2.   Composition and properties of high fibre diets.

gastric emptying [25], but there is a little evidence to suggest that viscous components tend to slow emptying [26].

Small Intestinal Effects

The cell wall material passes into the small intestine as fragments of plant tissue, and at this stage is completely hydrated, with the exception of the hydrophobic lignified regions and cutinised and suberised tissue. Some soluble components will increase the viscosity, and these affect diffusion of materials within the bulk contents and increase the "unstirred" layer at the mucosal surface [27]; this slows the rate of transport of water-soluble nutrients across the mucosal wall. In vitro studies show that these polysaccharides also alter mixed micelles. While binding of bile salts can also be demonstrated for a range of dietary fibre preparations in vitro, effects in vivo are more difficult to demonstrate. However, some malabsorption of fat does follow ingestion of some types of dietary fibre [28].

As digestion proceeds the polysaccharides of dietary fibre become the major carbohydrate components of the contents, together with the starch trapped within cellular structures and enzymatically resistant starch [29]. Associated with this mixture are proteins, inorganic materials, bile salts, and residual amounts of unabsorbed amino acids, fats and particularly salts of fatty acids. The mixture forms the material entering the large bowel. Direct analyses of this mixture are difficult to make, but ileostomy effluents provide some indicators [30] (Table 7.5).

Large Bowel Effects

The amount of dietary fibre ingested is a major contributor to the organic matter entering the large bowel. High fibre diets therefore increase the mass of material in the large intestine [31]. Many of the non-starch polysaccharides have water-binding properties [32] and thus increase both the dry matter and water contents in the proximal large intestine. Evidence for direct effects on large intestinal motility and pressures is somewhat equivocal [33], but the presence of bulk is believed to influence motility by acting on stretch-receptors [34].

One major role of the non-starch polysaccharides in the large bowel is the provision of substrates for the microflora [31], and these, together with unabsorbed sugars and undigested starch, are major sources of energy for the microflora, producing short-chain fatty acids (butyrate, acetate, propionate), carbon dioxide and hydrogen together with some methane [35]. The proportions of the different fatty acids formed are dependent on the types of polysaccharide being fermented, starch [36] producing more acetate and butyrate, whereas xylans and pectin produce mainly acetate, and arabinogalactans produce similar amounts of acetate and propionate. The polyphenolic materials in the cell wall modify the properties of the wall polysaccharides and tend to make the cell wall polysaccharides less readily degraded [37].

The dietary fibre not degraded by the microflora, together with the bacterial cell material, make up the major components of the faecal dry matter, so that increased excretion of organic matter is a characteristic of high fibre diets. The effects on faecal mass are dependent on the composition of the dietary fibre ingested, and, in general, less well fermented materials produce more faecal mass [31]. Faecal water concentra-

Table 7.5.   Effects of supplements of wheat bran and citrus pectin on the composition of ileostomy effluent (g or mmol/24 l)

		Wet weight[a] (g)	Dry matter[a] (g)	Ash[a] (g)	Organic matter[a] (g)	Total nitrogen (g)	Fat (+fatty acids)[a] (g)	Sodium[a] (mmol)	Potassium[a] (mmol)
Bran 16 g/day per head = 4.9 g DF[a]	Control	336	32	5.3	26.7	1.9	–	35	3.4
	Supplemented	457	41	6.6	34.4	2.0	–	46	3.8
Citrus pectin	Control	838	53	15.3	37.7	2.7[b]	9.4	84	7.0
15 g/day per head = 15 g DF	Supplemented	1152	77	20.3	56.7	3.5[b]	18.1	90	8.4
	Control	933	58	15.9	42.1	2.9[b]	8.4	126	11.2

Source: Sandberg et al. [30].
[a] DF, dietary fibre.
[b] Supplementation significantly altered excretion.
Analytical recovery of dietary fibre was virtually complete.

tion shows a relatively small increase but absolute losses of water via the faeces are greatly increased because of increased faecal mass. Some increased excretion of bile salts has been observed but the effects are dependent on the type of fibre fed [28].

The composition of the faecal flora is often characteristic of the individual, and studies of changes in the organisms present due to dietary fibre ingestion are somewhat equivocal [38,39]. There is some evidence of changes in bacterial enzymatic activities and studies using in vitro assessments of mutagenic activity suggest that the production of faecal mutagens is reduced on high fibre diets.

A large range of minor components of the diet that are unassimilable are effectively concentrated during passage through the gut, as more than 90% of the organic solids ingested are customarily digested and absorbed. These include many pigments, food colours, and traces of mineral oils [40]. The presence of dietary fibre dilutes the contents of the large bowel. Transit times are usually reduced by dietary fibre (41), but there are other powerful non-dietary determinants of transit time, and especially of large bowel residence times [42].

As well as the undegraded dietary fibre, increased faecal excretion of other dietary components if often observed [43] and increased dietary fibre intake effectively reduces the apparent digestibility of protein and lipids in the diet thus reducing the available (metabolisable) energy of the diet [44]. The effects are closely related to dietary fibre intake [45]. For the range of daily intake seen in the United Kingdom (15–40 g) the effects on total energy provision by the diet are relatively minor. The short-chain fatty acids produced by fermentation contribute energy to the body, but with UK intakes the contribution is minor and dependent on the amount and fermentability of the dietary fibre ingested [20]. Furthermore, there is evidence from animals of reduced efficiency of fat deposition from some dietary fibre sources [46]. However, the position with very high intakes (of the order of 100 g a day) is unknown, but may be significant in dietaries in developing countries.

Relation between the Physiological Effects of Dietary Fibre and Diseases of Affluence

It is important to bear in mind that the dietary fibre hypothesis [47,19] relates to a type of diet and studies are rare in which dietary fibre is the sole, or occasionally even the most important, dietary change. The epidemiology is further constrained by the inadequacies of quantitative data for the dietary fibre intakes of different populations. Data on food intake are inadequate, and dietary fibre is difficult to measure [8,10].

Obesity

In the early papers on the dietary fibre hypothesis [47] Trowell argued that, during his clinical career in Africa, he saw no obesity amongst rural populations living on an unrefined diet where the natural foods contained their fibre intact. Obesity only developed in the privileged urban population who had adopted a Westernised diet. Cleave [48] had held similar views and Heaton [49] presented a hypothesis that dietary fibre was protective against obesity because is surrounded the soluble sugars and starch in plant foods, and the structure of the natural unprocessed foods produced an early satiety effect, thus limiting voluntary food intake. It is possible to reject the quasi-epidemiological observations of the incidence of obesity as reflecting the effects of a low supply of food energy [50].

If dietary fibre has a role to play other than being a useful part of reduced energy diets [51] a mechanism of action has to be established. Three major types of mechanism have been proposed: (1) an effect on voluntary food intake: (2) an effect on the digestibility of the dietary energy; and (3) metabolic effects affecting satiety and the efficiency with which absorbed nutrients are utilised [52].

Effects on Voluntary Food Intake

The effect of dietary fibre on voluntary food intake rests on the hypothesis that less of a diet rich in dietary fibre will be consumed. This does assume that obesity can be regarded naively as being solely due to overeating, but nevertheless since obesity can only arise when food energy intake is in excess of expenditure [51] any dietary feature that acts to modulate energy intake would be expected to be associated with the aetiology of obesity.

Controlled experimental studies in man are virtually impossible to perform. There is some evidence to show an effect of dietary bulk in children [53] and studies of Heaton and his colleagues indicate that voluntary intake is reduced on a high fibre diet. During the studies of Southgate and Durnin [44], when diet was partially controlled, female subjects on the highest level of fibre intake (30 g/day) found the total amount of food difficult to eat.

Effects on Apparent Digestibility

The increased faecal energy loss associated with high fibre diets [44,54] at UK levels of intake is very small and cannot be regarded as a major effect of dietary fibre in the control of energy balance.

Metabolic Effects

Increased satiety has been demonstrated in some studies although the precise mechanism is not understood and the reduced glycaemic and insulinogenetic response to some types of dietary fibre may prove to be more significant [55]. It has been postulated that the tendency of dietary fibre to delay nutrient absorption and especially to produce some fat malabsorption may act through the "ileal brake" concept [56], and by a hormonal feedback on gastric emptying may act on satiety.

Direct metabolic effects of fibre ingestion are most likely to arise by two major routes: first by their effects on insulin secretion that may limit lipogenesis, and secondly by the effects of short-chain fatty acids on lipid metabolism. But at the present time these effects are hypothetical and await experimental testing.

The observations of Livesey and Davies [46] suggest that the fermentable non-starch polysaccharides may reduce fat deposition, and require detailed metabolic exploration.

Diabetes Mellitus

There is little reason to regard insulin-dependent diabetes mellitus (IDDM) as a disease of affluence, but the non-insulin-dependent condition (NIDDM) does show a low incidence in rural peasant communities and a higher incidence in developed communities [57]; and a very high incidence of the disease is seen in some isolated communities that could scarcely be considered affluent by worldwide standards. Trowell [58], on the basis of observations in communities in Africa, states that the condition developed when foods rich in refined carbohydrate became part of the diet, arguing that the separation of sugars and starches from the cell wall material in foods was a causative factor.

Many detailed studies have failed to show a demonstrable association between the consumption of sucrose and diabetes [59], and claims that changes in the intake of dietary fibre in the United Kingdom during World War II were associated chronologically with the decline in diabetes appear to be difficult to establish. Nevertheless, the close association between obesity and NIDDM may reveal indirect links between dietary fibre intakes and the disease. The high incidence in some communities has been claimed to be due to an increase in the overall availability of food after a very long period of relative deficiency of food which may have selected so-called thrifty populations. The association between obesity and insulin resistance and hyperinsulinaemia could be associated, albeit tenuously, with the effects of dietary fibre on rates of glucose absorption and insulin secretion, associated with viscous non-starch polysaccharides and foods where cellular structures have not been destroyed. Anthropological evidence [60] on the early development of the human diet indicates that before the development of cereal cultivation early man would have consumed substantial amounts of polysaccharides from fruits and vegetables. Such diets would have slow glycaemic characteristics. Without a direct understanding of the aetiology of NIDDM, the precise role of dietary fibre will remain unclear. However, increased dietary fibre from a variety of sources within a diet that is low in fat, and with most of the available carbohydrate as complex carbohydrates, has major benefits in the management of many cases of NIDDM [61].

Coronary Heart Disease

Long-term epidemiological studies have shown that men with highest intakes of dietary fibre had the lowest experience of coronary heart disease (CHD) [68].

Deaths from cardiovascular disease, especially amongst men aged 45–60, are highest in countries where living standards are high. The distribution of cerebrovascular disease tends to be less closely related to the standard of living [62]. A link between ischaemic heart disease and dietary fibre intake was postulated by Trowell [63]. The evidence was primarily epidemiological, in particular the extremely low prevalence of the disease in rural African populations. Initially, attention was focussed on the possible link with one of the major risk factors, serum cholesterol levels, because these are low in rural African populations and also amongst vegetarian groups (which have higher dietary fibre intakes than the remainder of the population).

The mechanism of action postulated was that the binding of bile salts to dietary fibre, and their excretion in faeces, prevented their recycling and that the increased rates of synthesis would deplete the cholesterol pool [64]. Despite the clear evidence of in vitro binding of bile salts, the mechanism whereby dietary fibre, in particular the more soluble viscous polysaccharide components, lowers cholesterol is not clearly established [65]. Effects on blood lipids can also be seen in reduced low density lipoprotein cholesterol components [66].

The true significance of dietary fibre in the context of the diet is confounded by the fact that fat intake as a proportion of total energy intake is not independent of carbohydrate intake [15], and that both saturated fat and cholesterol intakes tend to be negatively associated with dietary fibre intakes [67] in free-living subjects.

Large Bowel Disease

The benefits of an increased intake of dietary fibre in large bowel disease were amongst the first protective effects to be postulated [4]. For the purposes of the present discussion it is convenient to consider these disease states in two categories: intra-abdominal "pressure diseases" and large bowel cancer. The former include a range of conditions such as diverticular disease, varicose veins, haemorrhoids, appendicitis and hiatus hernia.

Pressure Diseases

In pressure diseases the effects of low intakes of dietary fibre are regarded as causative. Thus Painter and Burkitt [4] postulated that diverticular disease was a deficiency disease due to low intake of dietary fibre. The epidemiological evidence was firstly that the incidence of the condition in rural Africans was low although the urban black populations in the United States showed a similar incidence to the whites. Furthermore Burkitt argued that in the United Kingdom diverticular disease was unknown in the early part of the century until the consumption of cereals, potatoes and other vegetables declined. The postulated mechanism was that a low intake of fibre led to reduced mass in the large bowel, with a consequently prolonged period for fermentation and water reabsorption, leading to low viscous/solid contents which in turn demanded a high propulsive contraction pressure. This led to segmentation and herniation of the bowel wall [4]. Treatment of diverticulitis with high fibre diets produced symptomatic relief in many patients and reduced the need for surgery [69].

Subsequent studies of pressures developed in the large bowel tended to support the aetiological concept, but some bulk laxatives did not appear to reduce pressures despite some symptomatic relief [33]. Studies with wheat bran preparations have tended to dominate this area and Brodribb [70] showed that particle size was important, possibly because large particulate bran was less well fermented and therefore increased bulk more effectively. Many studies of this topic have not had adequate dietary control and dose–response effects have been decidedly equivocal. The postulated long exposure to a low fibre diet required for the development of the condition makes retrospective studies extremely difficult to perform. Long-term studies with rats [71] fed on different levels of cereal dietary fibre show quite conclusively that low fibre intakes do produce extensive diverticular disease in rats.

Evidence for association of a low fibre diet with the range of other pressure diseases is primarily epidemiological. While the aetiology is unclear it is postulated that straining at stool is involved when the faecal mass is hard and dry, as is characteristic of a low fibre diet [72].

Large Bowel Cancer

The aetiological observations which led to the hypothesis that dietary fibre protects against large bowel cancer stem from Burkitt [73]. Since then a number of more detailed studies have been inconclusive. In part this was due to deficiencies in dietary intake data [74]. Detailed studies where direct measurements of dietary fibre were made [75,76] suggest that there was evidence for a protective effect of non-starch polysaccharides. The mechanisms invoked include the effects of dietary fibre on faecal bulk, transit time, pH, bacterial metabolism and alterations in the production of mutagens.

Cummings [74] argues that without a sound understanding of the aetiology of large bowel cancer, the significance of the established effects of dietary fibre on the physiology of the large bowel is difficult to assess. It is difficult to envisage a pathogenesis in which a low fibre intake is itself causative and it may well be that a low intake provides a colonic environment where other more directly carcinogenic agents can act, and that dietary fibre may protect. Studies with chemical carcinogens and dietary fibre have given conflicting results, and at the present time the direct link with dietary fibre intake is best regarded as plausible but unproven [77]. It is also probable that, again, a high dietary fibre intake is an indicator of a diet with lower levels of other dietary risk factors such as fat and animal protein [78], and higher levels of vegetable consumption which may be associated with other naturally occurring anticarcinogenic agents [79].

Conclusions

From the foregoing account it is clear that many components of dietary fibre exert physiological effects that are due to the range of chemical structures, physical properties and physical structures that the term dietary fibre embraces. These physiological effects can be related to the aetiology of some diseases but in most cases the diseases are strictly of unknown aetiology and therefore direct links to the physiological effects of dietary fibre are not possible at the present time.

Epidemiological studies where dietary fibre intakes have been related to disease incidence produce equivocal weak correlations in multivariate statistical analysis, and variations in dietary fibre intake account for only part of the variation in incidence. Thus direct links between the diseases and dietary fibre *per se* cannot be established. In part the weak relationships are due to a lack of satisfactory data for dietary fibre intakes in many, if not all population groups. This is primarily due to one of the major weaknesses of current nutritional science – the measurement of food intake in free-living subjects [80,81] – coupled with a lack of comprehensive data on the dietary fibre in foods.

No epidemiological studies have yet refuted the central hypothesis of protective effects, and similarly most of the physiological effects of dietary fibre that have been established are also compatible with the hypothesis. At the same time it must be recognised that few sources of dietary fibre have been the subject of critical study in man. Much of the evidence points to dietary fibre in the context of the diet, in other words the effects on a disease incidence seem to be more likely to be related to the type of diet rather than one component. The central issue is therefore to consider how this relationship can be explored scientifically, and how the integrated concept of a balanced diet can be presented. A formal treatment of how this issue could be described is given in the Appendix.

Desirable Levels of Dietary Fibre

In the absence of a formal relationship between any one disease and dietary intake, any quantitative recommendation for dietary fibre intakes is difficult to sustain. This is further confounded by the heterogeneity of dietary fibre itself, so that any quantitative definition of dietary intakes would need to define the actual composition of the dietary fibre. There are two possible approaches. The first of these is to select the one physiological effect where there is a little evidence on dose-related effects: normalisation of colonic function to bring mean turnover time [82] into the region of 45 hours and faecal wet weight to around 100–150 g/day. On the basis of a range of bulking studies [41] with a group of young men the requirement for this is approximately 30 g/day per head of dietary fibre from mixed sources. These observations formed the basis of the NACNE [2] recommendations, and was based on intakes measured by the Southgate [11] method, which includes resistant starch and lignins. In non-starch polysaccharide [29] terms this is equivalent to about 21 g/day per head.

At present it is unclear whether the amount of dietary fibre required to normalise colonic function is an absolute value or whether it is a function of body size or energy intake. These uncertainties make the formulation of recommendations for women and children with lower body size and energy intakes, or the elderly with low energy intakes, difficult, because an absolute requirement demands the consumption of diets with different dietary fibre/energy densities (Fig. 7.3) and this has implications for the mixture of foods to be consumed (Fig. 7.4). The recommended intakes should probably be related to body size.

The second approach is to construct diets that meet the compositional requirements in respect of the dietary risk factors that are more securely based. Thus, reducing the proportion of energy from fat in the diet will increase the carbohydrate intake. If at the same time sucrose intakes are not increased, and possibly reduced, following the recommendations of the Royal College of Physicians' report on obesity [51], these dietary changes will generate higher fibre intakes that, on the basis of limited dietary modelling calculations [83], would produce dietary fibre intakes in the range suggested by NACNE.

Summary

Dietary fibre is a mixture of polysaccharides with different chemical and physical properties. It is therefore not possible to generalise about the effects of dietary fibre intakes. Most of the established physiological effects of dietary fibre are consistent with the protective hypothesis.

The protective effects of high fibre diets are, however, most probably due to properties of the diets themselves in addition to the specific effects of the dietary fibre they contain.

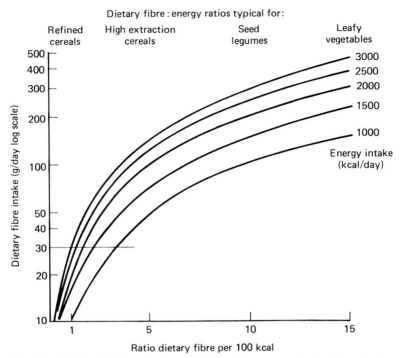

Fig. 7.3. Relationship between the ratio dietary fibre : energy in the diet to intake of dietary fibre at different total energy intakes. The figure shows that in order to achieve intakes of 30 g/day diets with different nutrient densities (g dietary fibre/100 kcal) are required for different levels of energy intake. Thus at 2500 kcal/day a density of 1.2 g/100 kcal is required, while at 1000 kcal/day the required density is 3.0 g/100 kcal.

Appendix. Towards a Formal Analysis of the Relation Between Diet and Health/Disease

The proposition is that "health" is a function of the composition of the dietary intake. In formal terms the corollary of this is that some dietary change will be associated with a change in health.

While it is not possible, for reasons that will become apparent below, to define the form that the function takes, it is useful to consider what the characteristics of the function might be, and what experimental measurements could be designed to test the central proposition.

It is clear that at the limits – no, or very low food intakes, and vastly excessive food intakes – health is certainly a function of dietary intake and that the relation is an inverted U.

The first essential in establishing the function is to define the dependent variable "health". In most acceptable definitions health is a positive and integrated state involving both physical and psychological well-being, and for the purposes of the proposition is undefinable in quantitative terms that would permit the evaluation of

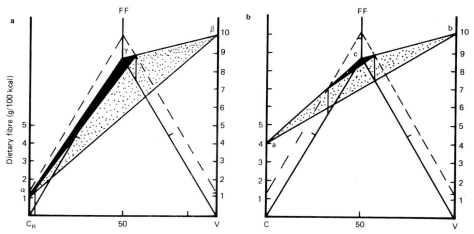

Fig. 7.4a,b.   Dietary fibre : energy ratios in dietary mixtures. **a** In this three-dimensional figure the triangle CR,V,FF contains all mixtures of refined cereals, vegetables and fibre-free components. The vertical axes are dietary fibre : energy (g/100 kcal) ratios. The plane surface α,β,γ contains all possible ratios; the *black* area represents those mixtures below 1.2 g/100 kcal. The figure shows that a diet with refined cereal cannot achieve this ratio even at 100% of energy from cereal. Some vegetables must be present with a limit of 13–3%, the latter requiring 97% of energy from cereals, i.e. *no* fibre-free foods at all.

b In this figure the dietary fibre ratios of all mixtures of whole extraction cereals, vegetables and fibre-free foods are contained in the plane a,b,c. The limits of the diets below 1.2 g dietary fibre per 100 kcal (the *black* region) are 35% cereal and 13% vegetables as percentage of energy. The figure shows that a much wider range of dietary mixtures have dietary fibre : energy ratios above 1.2 g/100 kcal when high extraction cereals are part of the diet.

the function. Health is clearly not merely the absence of disease, nor can it be thought of as the reciprocal of disease incidence. Likewise indicators such as life expectancy, infant mortality or death from coronary heart disease (CHD) are not true measures of health, although reports such as those of NACNE [2] and COMA have been translated in these terms. Thus a dietary change that it is predicted will reduce CHD deaths is interpreted as a healthy change, whereas in strict terms it is a disease preventive measure: a public health measure. Since it is not possible to define the dependent variable in quantitative terms, it is impossible to derive or test the initial proposition, which must therefore be modified to "The incidence of a disease is a function of dietary intake". In other words some change in diet will produce a change in the incidence of a disease. Clearly such a relation with infective disease is likely to be weak, although a dietary interaction is likely in some, if not many instances. Disease incidence in these cases is more commonly a function of the prevalance of the infective agent and the inherent resistance of the population. If we consider a disease of unknown aetiology, where there is presumptive evidence for a dietary factor, we can examine the relation between incidence and dietary composition; and from this we can establish the function that relates diet to incidence, because incidence is quantifiable.

Using cardiovascular disease as an example, death from ischaemic heart disease is usually associated with a thrombotic incident which obstructs the coronary vessels. Such an episode is a chance event, precipitated by a number of factors, many of which are unrelated to the diet being eaten immediately before the event. The predisposing condition is the presence of lesions in the arterial wall and the accumulation of plaques, the chance detachment of which precipitates the incident. The lesions in the arterial wall develop with time, and are probably related *inter alia* to dietary factors. Thus it is the incidence of ischaemic arterial disease, not the thrombotic incident, that is most likely to be involved. If deaths from CHD are closely related to the prevalence and severity of arterial changes, then it may be valid to use deaths as the measured dependent variable. If they are not, then there is little reason to expect the incidence of deaths from CHD to be a function of diet. Furthermore, since the formation of the arterial lesions is time-dependent it is reasonable to expect the incidence of atheroma to be a function that integrates the diet consumed over a period of time.

A further factor that must be considered is that the incidence of deaths from CHD in the population as a whole will include those from individuals with lipidaemias who may be genetically predisposed, and those from older members of the population of age greater than say, 70 years. It is thus desirable to limit examination of incidence to a defined population, say, between 40 and 60 years.

At this stage one can draw a number of conclusions.

1. Relationship between health *sensu stricto* and diet cannot be defined or tested.
2. A relationship between disease incidence and diet could establish a rationale for disease prevention by dietary means.
3. The dietary function will almost certainly be an integration of diet over a period of time.
4. Since deaths from a disease are not necessarily a measure of incidence, the relation between deaths and diet cannot be expected to be strong, unless a specific dietary constituent acts as a causative agent, i.e. behaves as a toxin.

The dietary intake term could be expressed in terms of dietary composition *per se*, implying a relationship that is independent of the amounts consumed or in terms of amounts consumed. It is common practice to express consumption on a compositional basis, such as percentage of total energy consumption, or per 100 kcal, in order to facilitate comparisons between individuals with very different total food intakes. This appears to make the implicit assumption that it is dietary composition rather than absolute intake that is part of the relation between disease incidence and diet.

The composition of a diet containing n constituents can be expressed in terms of $n-1$ dimensions. The relation between disease incidence and diet therefore relates to a variable that is expressed as a domain in $n-1$ dimensions. Many of the dimensions are not independent, and many dimensions are constrained by the nature of foods and dietary choice, so that extremes of the range are seen in very few individuals. If dietary intake is expressed in terms of energy then it is possible to establish some preliminary features of the dietary composition of domains.

Firstly, protein, although variable in composition in respect of both amino acid and tertiary protein structures, is a variable with a very restricted range when expressed as percentage of energy intake, and for the purposes of the present discussion can be considered constant at about 10% of the energy intake. The first dimension, therefore, may be percentage energy from fat. However, in the classical proximate view of diet, with protein held constant, fat energy and carbohydrate energy are not independent, so that the first dimension has the limits 90% fat energy and 90% carbohydrate energy, the usual range lying between 10% and 50% fat energy (80% carbohydrate and 40% carbohydrate).

A second dimension, not necessarily perpendicular to the first, is the proportion of carbohydrate consumed as free sugars. Diets may range from carbohydrate mixtures

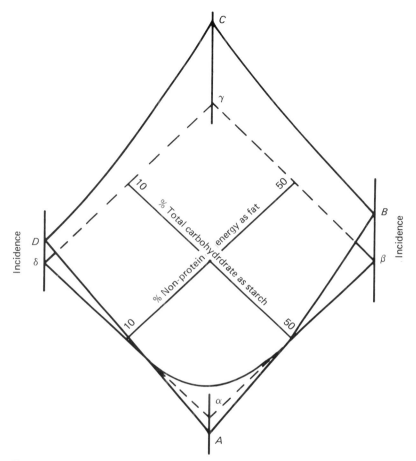

Fig. A.1. Hypothetical representation of an incidence surface with dietary composition varying in two dimensions. Incidence at all dietary compositions lies on the surface $ABCD$. This is based on the assumption that there is a weak link between incidence and proportion of energy from fat. The rectangle $\alpha\beta\gamma\delta$ represents a surface where there is no link between diet and incidence.

where sugar and starch intakes are approximately equal, to those where starch is greatly in excess of sugar. This provides four major domains.

A third dimension, again not necessarily perpendicular to the first or second, may be taken as the fat composition, which can be expressed in terms of a ratio of polyunsaturated to saturated fats (P : S). Although the theoretical limits are 0 to infinity, in practice the range is from 0 to 1. This provides eight domains. Extension to other dimensions, such as dietary fibre composition, protein source and other nutrients, cannot be represented physically.

Dietary composition can also be defined in terms of food. Here the numbers of components could be of the order of 10^5, if foods are described precisely according to proprietary brands, type of cooking and processing procedure. Since the types and amounts of food define the composition of the diet in the nutrient components domains, it is clear that the movements in these domains in response to dietary changes in foods selected for consumption are extremely complex. This is possibly a major reason why the relationships between disease incidence and the consumption of individual foods are weak and ill-defined, unless a toxic constituent or microbial contaminant is implicated.

At this point it is possible to draw some further conclusions:

1. The function relating dietary intake to disease incidence must recognise that dietary intake is delineated within a multidimensional domain, and the possibility that a *simple* relationship exists must be rejected.
2. The compositional domain is defined by the amounts and precise types of food eaten and cannot be *precisely defined* in free-living communities with existing techniques.

If we limit the dimensions in which diet is defined to two, then we can postulate that incidence will approach a minimum when composition is optimal. Since diet is variable over two dimensions incidence is represented as a surface (see Fig. A.1).

Dietary changes will move the composition of the diet in any direction, and the change in incidence will move over the surface. However, any dietary change involving changes in foods eaten will rarely be parallel to any one dimension.

This implies that dietary recommendations should be couched in terms that avoid presenting any one food or groups of foods as desirable or undesirable or focussing on specific nutrients, because the reality is infinitely more complex than the figure indicates. It may well be that a return to the concept of balancing intake of the major food groups is the most sound approach.

References

1. Sherman HC (1933) Chemistry of food and nutrition, 4th ed. Macmillan, New York
2. Health Education Council (1983) Proposals for nutrition guidelines for health education in Britain. National Advisory Committee for Nutrition Education, London
3. Health and welfare in Canada (1985) Report of the Expert Advisory Committee on Dietary Fibre. Ministry of National Health and Welfare, Ottawa
4. Painter NS, Burkitt DP (1971) Diverticular disease of the colon: a deficiency disease of Western civilization. Br Med J ii:450–454
5. Hipsley EH (1953) Dietary "fibre" and pregnancy toxaemia. Br Med J ii:420–422
6. Trowell H, Southgate DAT, Wolever TMS, Leeds AR, Gassul MA, Jenkins DJA (1976) Dietary fibre redefined. Lancet I:967
7. Southgate DAT, Hudson GJ, Englyst H (1978) The analysis of dietary fibre, the choices for the analyst. J Sci Food Agric 29:979–988
8. Southgate DAT, Englyst HN (1985) Dietary fibre: chemistry, physical properties and analysis. In: Trowell H, Burkitt D, Heaton K (eds) Dietary fibre, fibre depleted foods and disease. Academic Press, London pp 31–55
9. Southgate DAT (1988) Lignin a part of the dietary fibre complex? Proceedings of Kelloggs symposium 1987. John Libbey, London (in press)
10. Selvendran RR, Du Pont MS (1984) The analysis of dietary fibre. In: King R (ed) Food analysis techniques, vol 3. Applied Science Publishers, London, pp 1–68
11. Southgate DAT (1969) Determination of carbohydrates in foods. II. Unavailable carbohydrates. J Sci Food Agric 20:331–335
12. Southgate DAT (1976) Determination of food carbohydrates. Applied Science Publishers, London
13. Burkitt DP, Trowell HC (eds) (1975) Refined carbohydrate foods and disease. Some implications of dietary fibre. Academic Press, New York
14. Whitehead M (1987) The health divide: inequalities in health in the 1980s. Health Education Council, London

15. Perisse J, Sizaret F, Francois P (1969) The effect of income on the structure of the diet. FAO Nutrition Newsletter 7. FAO, Rome, pp 1–9
16. FAO/WHO (1980) Carbohydrates in human nutrition. Food and Nutrition Paper 15. FAO, Rome
17. Southgate DAT (1987) Minerals, trace elements and potential hazards. J Am Clin Nutr 45:1256–1266
18. Wahlquist ML, Jones GP, Hansky J, Duncan SD, Coles-Rutishauser I, Littlejohn GO (1981) The role of dietary fibre in human health. Food Technol Aust 35:51–52
19. Southgate DAT, Penson JM (1983) Testing the dietary fibre hypothesis. In: Birch GG, Parker JJ (eds) Dietary fibre. Applied Science Publishers, London, pp 1–19
20. Southgate DAT (1976) The chemistry of dietary fiber. In: Spiller GA, Amen RJ (eds) Fiber in human nutrition. Plenum Press, New York, pp 31–72
21. Selvendran RR (1984) The plant cell wall as a source of dietary fibre: chemistry and structure. J Clin Nutr 39:320–327
22. Southgate DAT (1986) Food components associated with dietary fiber. In: Spiller GA (ed) Handbook of dietary fiber in human nutrition. CRC Press, Boca Raton, pp 23–26
23. Southgate DAT (1980) Characteristics of dietary fiber. Rep Int Assoc Cereal Chem 10:79–81
24. Mitchell AN, Southgate DAT (1969) Observation on the passage of food through the gastro-intestinal tract of the rat. Proc Nutr Soc 28:7 (abstract)
25. Read NW, Miles CA, Fisher D et al. (1980) Transit of a meal through the stomach, small intestine and colon in normal subjects and its role in the pathogenesis of diarrhoea. Gasteroenterology 79:1276–1282
26. Holt S, Heading RC, Carter DC, Prescott LF, Tothill P (1979) Effect of gel fibre on gastric emptying and absorption of glucose and paracetamol. Lancet I:636–639
27. Johnson IT, Gee JM (1981) Effect of gel forming gums on the intestinal unstirred layer and sugar transport in vitro. Gut 22:398–403
28. Story JA, Kritchevsky D (1976) Comparison of the binding of the various bile acids and bile salts in vitro by several different types of fiber. J Nutr 106:1292–1294
29. Englyst HN, Cummings JH (1987) Resistant starch, a "new" food component: a classification of starch for nutritional purposes. In: Morton ID (ed) Cereals in a European context. Ellis Horwood, Chichester
30. Sandberg AS, Andersson H, Hallgren B, Hasselblad K, Isaksson B, Hulten L (1981) Experimental model for in vivo determination of dietary fibre and its effects on the absorption of nutrients in the small intestine. Br J Nutr 45:283–294
31. Stephen AM, Cummings JH (1980) Mechanism of action of dietary fibre in the human colon. Nature 284:283–284
32. McConnell AA, Eastwood MA, Mitchell WD (1974) Physical characteristics of vegetable foodstuffs that could influence bowel function. J Sci Food Agric 25:1457–1464
33. Eastwood MA, Smith AN, Brydon WG, Pritchard J (1978) Comparison of bran, ispaghula and lactulose on colonic function in diverticular disease. Gut 19:1144–1147
34. Truelove SC (1966) Movements of the large intestine. Physiol Rev 46:457–512
35. Cummings JH (1981) Short chain fatty acids in the human colon. Gut 22: 763–779
36. Englyst HN, Hay S, Macfarlane GT (1987) Polysaccharide breakdown by mixed populations of human gut bacteria. Microb Ecol 95:163–171
37. Selvendran RR (1987) Chemistry of plant cell walls and dietary fibre. Scand J Gastroenterol 22:33–41
38. Bornside GE (1978) Stability of human fecal flora. Am J Clin Nutr 31 (Suppl):141–144
39. Drasar BS, Hill MJ (1972) Intestinal bacteria and cancer. Am J Clin Nutr 25:1399–1404
40. Southgate DAT (1973) Non-assimilable components of foods. In: Hollingsworth DF, Russell M (eds) Nutritional problems in a changing world. Applied Science Publishers, London, pp 199–204
41. Cummings JH, Southgate DAT, Branch W, Houston H, Jenkins DJA, James WPT (1978) Colonic response to dietary fibre from carrot, cabbage, apple bran and guar gum. Lancet I:5–9
42. Avery Jones F, Godding EW (1972) Management of constipation. Blackwell Scientific Publications, Oxford
43. Southgate DAT (1986) Digestion and absorption of nutrients. In: Vahouney GA, Kritchevsky D (eds) Dietary fibre in health and disease. Plenum Press, New York, pp 45–52
44. Southgate DAT, Durnin JVGA (1970) Calorie conversion factors, an experimental re-assessment of the factors used in the calculation of the energy value of human diets. Br J Nutr 24:517–535
45. Southgate DAT (1975) Fibre and other unavailable carbohydrates and energy effects in the diet. In: White PL, Selvey N (eds) Proceedings of Western Hemisphere nutrition congress IV. Acton Mass. Publishing Sciences Group, Acton, Mass., pp 51–55
46. Davies IR, Johnson IT, Livesey G (1987) Food energy values of dietary fibre components and decreased deposition of body fat. Int J Obes 11 (Suppl I):101–115

47. Trowell H (1976) Definition of dietary fiber and hypotheses that it is a protective factor in certain diseases. Am J Clin Nutr 29:417–427
48. Cleave TL (1974) The saccharine disease. Wright, Bristol
49. Heaton KW (1973) Food fibre as an obstacle to energy intake. Lancet II:1418–1421
50. FAO (annually) Provisional food balance sheets. FAO, Rome
51. Royal College of Physicians (1983) Obesity. J R Coll Physicians Lond 17:3–58
52. Southgate DAT (1978) Has dietary fibre a role in the prevention and treatment of obesity? Bibl Nutr Dieta 26:70–76
53. Rutishauser IHE, Whitehead RG (1972) Energy intake and expenditure in 1–3 year old Ugandan children living in a rural environment. Br J Nutr 28:145–152
54. McNeil NI (1984) The contribution of the large intestine to energy supplied in man. Am J Clin Nutr 39:338–342
55. Smith U (1987) Dietary fibre, diabetes and obesity. Scand J Gastroenterol 22 (Suppl 129):151–153
56. Welch I, Saunders K, Read NW (1985) Effects of ileal and intravenous infusions of fat emulsions on feeding and satiety in human volunteers. Gastroenterology 89:1293–1297
57. Zimmet P (1982) Type 2 (non-insulin dependent) diabetes: an epidemiological overview. Diabetologia 22:399–411
58. Trowell HC (1973) Dietary fibre, coronary heart disease and diabetes mellitus. Plant Foods for Man 1:11–16
59. Sugars Task Force (1986) Evaluation of health aspects of sugars contained in carbohydrate sweeteners. J Nutr 116 (Suppl):11
60. Eaton SB, Konner M (1985) Paleolithic nutrition. A consideration of its nature and current implications. N Engl J Med 312:283–289
61. Mann J (1985) Diabetes mellitus: some aspects of the aetiology and management of non-insulin dependent diabetes. In: Trowell H, Burkitt D, Heaton K (eds) Dietary fibre, fibre-depleted foods and disease. Academic Press, New York pp 263–287
62. Junge B, Hoffmeister H (1982) Civilization associated diseases in Europe and industrial countries outside of Europe: regional differences and trends in mortality. Prev Med 11:117–130
63. Trowell H (1972) Ischemic heart disease and dietary fiber. Am J Clin Nutr 962–932
64. Pyorala K (1987) Dietary cholesterol in relation to plasma cholesterol and coronary heart disease. Am J Clin Nutr 45:1176–1184
65. Story JA, Lord SL (1987) Bile salts: in vitro studies with fibre components. Scand J Gastroenterol 22:174–80
66. Miettinen TA (1987) Dietary fiber and lipids. Am J Clin Nutr 45:1237–1242
67. Neissen C, Brussard JH, Katan MB (1983) Serum lipiden en samenstelling van de voeding van 371 Wageningse studenten. Voeding 44:350–355
68. Morris JN, Marr JW, Clayton DG (1977) Diet and heart: a postscript. Br Med J ii:1307–1314
69. Cummings JH (1984) Constipation, dietary fibre and the control of large bowel function. Postgrad Med J 60:811–819
70. Brodribb AJM, Grove SC (1978) Effect of bran particle size in stool weight. Gut 19:60–63
71. Fisher N, Berry CS, Fearn T (1985) Cereal dietary fiber consumption and diverticular disease. Am J Clin Nutr 42:788–804
72. Burkitt DP (1985) Varicose veins, haemorrhoids, deep vein thrombosis and pelvic phleboliths. In: Trowell H, Burkitt DP, Heaton K (eds) Dietary fibre, fibre depleted foods and disease. Academic Press, New York pp 317–329
73. Burkitt DP (1971) Epidemiology of cancer of the colon and rectum. Cancer 28:3–13
74. Cummings J (1985) Cancer of the large bowel. In: Trowell H, Burkitt DP, Heaton K (eds) Dietary fibre, fibre depleted foods and disease. Academic Press, New York, pp 161–182.
75. International Agency for Research in Cancer Micro-ecology Group (1977) Dietary fibre, transit-time, faecal bacteria, steroids and colon cancer in two Scandinavian populations. Lancet II:207–211
76. Jensen OM, MacLennan R, Wahrendorf J (1982) Diet, bowel function, fecal characteristics and large bowel cancer in Denmark and Finland. Nutr Cancer 4:5–19
77. Mendeloff AI (1987) Dietary fiber and gastrointestinal disease. Am J Clin Nutr 45:1267–1270
78. Drasar BS, Irving D (1973) Environmental factors and cancers of the colon and breast. Br J Cancer 27:167–172
79. Wattenberg LW (1983) Inhibition of neoplasia by minor dietary constitutents. Cancer Res 43 (Suppl):2448–2453
80. Marr JW (1971) Individual dietary surveys: purposes and methods. Karger, Basel, pp 105–164 (World review of nutrition and dietetics vol 13)
81. Stockley L (1985) Changes in habitual food intake, during weighed inventory surveys and duplicate diet collections. A short review. Ecol Food Nutr 17:263–269

82. Cummings JH, Jenkins DJA, Wiggins HS (1976) Measurement of mean transit time of dietary residues through the gut of man. Gut 17:210–218
83. Robbins CJ (ed) (1978) Food, health and farming reports of panels on the implications for UK agriculture. Centre for Agricultural Strategy, Reading

Commentary

Jarrett: Southgate contrasts the dimensions of diets in affluent compared with developing countries, with the latter being characterised by low fat energy, high starch and low animal protein. Japan is a very affluent country which departs from the general rule. It is also a country whose population now has the greatest expectation of life at birth and low rates of coronary heart disease which are actually falling [1]. This is not a genetic advantage for migrant Japanese are not so favoured [2]. If the traditional Japanese cuisine is largely responsible for the longevity and relative freedom from coronary disease, it would repay some study. Apart from the high carbohydrate/low fat aspect, are there data on other dietary constituents such as fibre and micronutrients?

Trends in ischaemic heart disease mortality in Japan and changes in a number of other variables are discussed in a recent paper by Ueshima et al. [1]. In both sexes mortality rates have declined in the age groups 50–59 and 60–69 years since the late 1960s. These have occurred in the face of rising fat consumption and decreasing P : S ratios. No information is given on salt or fibre consumption. With regard to blood pressure, in national samples both diastolic and systolic pressures in both sexes increased from 1956 to 1964 and have decreased since 1964, though in men the average values were still higher in 1980 than in 1956. The authors thought that the reduction in blood pressure was due to more widespread hypotensive therapy. Although it does not explain the fall in mortality rates, it is worth noting that the National Cardiovascular Survey of 1980 reported average serum cholesterol levels in males age 50–59 years of only 189 mg/100 ml; in women it was 203 mg/100 ml [3]. Smoking rates differed very much between the sexes, with (in 1980) 70% of men smoking daily or occasionally compared with 14% of women. Despite these high smoking rates, mortality from all causes in men aged 45–64 years was almost halved between 1950 and 1978 [4], giving Japanese men easily the lowest mortality rates in the 26 selected countries. A similar fall occurred in Japanese women, but their rates were rivalled by women in Switzerland, Sweden and Norway.

The relevance of the foregoing to dietary fibre may be hard to discern, but it is intended to illustrate the problem of attempting to explain trends (in morbidity and mortality) by any univariate approach. (See my commentary on Chapter 5.)

References

1. Ueshima H, Tatara K, Asakura S (1987) Declining mortality from ischemic heart disease and changes in coronary risk factors in Japan, 1956–1980. Am J Epidemiol 125:62–72
2. Gordon T (1975) Mortality experience among the Japanese in the United States, Hawaii and Japan. Public Health Rep 72:543–553
3. Public Health Bureau, Ministry of Health and Welfare (1982) National survey on circulatory disorders, 1980. Japan Heart Foundation, Tokyo
4. Thom TJ, Epstein FH, Feldman JJ, Leaverton PE (1985) Trends in total mortality and mortality from heart disease in 26 countries from 1950 to 1978. Int J Epidemiol 14:510–520

Author's reply: It is true that Japan does appear to be an exception in having a low incidence of the diseases under discussion and a low dietary fibre intake. The Japanese diet is, however, rich in starch, and it is now recognised that a substantial amount of food starch is resistant to enzymatic hydrolysis in the small intestine. This resistant starch therefore passes into the large intestine where it is fermented by the intestinal microflora in a way that is strictly analogous to many components of dietary fibre in the plant cell wall sense.

It is becoming evident that the amount of in vivo enzymatically resistant starch may be greater than the intake of dietary fibre. The protective properties of high fibre diets may in part be due to the fact that they are high starch diets.

Thomas: Fibre in relation to society is of particular interest to those concerned with obesity and weight control. I would like to draw attention to a useful recent review in this field [1].

Reference

1. Blundell JE, Burley VJ (1987) Satiation, satiety and the action of fibre on food intake. Int J Obes 11 (Suppl 1):9–25

Sanders: The statement that high fibre diets have a low energy density and a low physical density is a common misconception. We have studied the growth and development of children reared on vegan diets. Although the energy intakes of the diets were low, this could not be attributed to a high consumption of fibre-rich foods. Indeed, it was cereals, nuts and pulses that provided most of the dietary energy. Where energy intakes were restricted this was due to the overconsumption of fruit and vegetables. Children allowed to choose freely will select the more energy-dense foods. Those foods which are regarded as the richest source of fibre, for example wholemeal bread, pulses (particularly soya beans) and nuts, are energy-dense foods. Diets containing high proportions of fruit and vegetables do tend to be bulky but do not make a great contribution to total fibre intake. There certainly appears to be a tendency to confuse bulk with fibre intake.

Author's reply: This is further evidence that the properties of high fibre diets are related not to fibre content *per se*, but to the properties of the foods.

Sanders: The suggestion that the high incidence of non-insulin-dependent diabetes mellitus (NIDDM) is due to selection of thrifty populations is illogical. NIDDM only becomes manifest in middle-age, often beyond reproductive age. Environmental selection can only act if individuals do not reach reproductive age.

Dietary fibre intake has not emerged as a risk factor for coronary heart disease; (CHD) in most prospective studies. The study of Marr (Southgate's reference 80) compared fibre intakes in bus conductors and drivers. The bus drivers had more CHD, lower energy intakes and were fatter than the conductors. It would be expected, therefore, that they would also have correspondingly lower fibre intakes. CHD mortality rates and the incidence of NIDDM are high amongst men of Indian descent. They have dietary intakes that correspond to those advocated by NACNE. Their intakes of dietary fibre are of the order of 28–30 g/day. The Japanese, who have a low incidence of CHD and NIDDM, have intakes of fibre comparable with the British average. Systematic studies have failed to show that wheat fibre intakes influence serum cholesterol, blood pressure or other haemostatic factors. Although certain soluble fibres, particularly guar gum and pectin, do lower plasma cholesterol concentrations and improve glucose tolerance, the intakes required are relatively high compared with what can be obtained from the diet. Health educators have unwisely extrapolated effects obtained with high doses of soluble fibre to low doses of all types of fibre.

Author's reply: The statistical analysis isolated the effect of energy intake, and a relation to fibre remained.

Chapter 8

Changing Lifestyles: The Effects on a Balanced Diet

J. E. Thomas

Introduction

In recent years it has become popular to characterise the group of conditions which includes cardiovascular disease, obesity, diabetes and dental caries as "diseases of Western civilisation", or diseases of affluence. This strongly suggests that the dietary component in the aetiology of such conditions is closely related to aspects of the lifestyle associated with a relatively affluent, largely industrialised society. Implicit in this proposition is the idea that humans have very poorly developed innate mechanisms for the regulation of energy and nutrient intake, mechanisms which would influence the selection of foods from those available in such a way as to ensure a balanced diet.

Migration studies are seen to have contributed greatly to the understanding of the epidemiology of such clinical conditions, and they appear to support the priority accorded to social and lifestyle factors in influencing food choice. In this instance, they appear to support the specific proposition that the characteristic features of an industrialised lifestyle influence food selection in a way which is likely to promote consumption of an "unbalanced" diet.

For the purposes of this paper, a balanced diet is taken to mean "a diet which prevents deficiency diseases and which sustains a healthy vigorous life. That is, a diet which contains all the essential nutrients in the optimum proportion for the individual" [1].

This paper will examine the role of innate mechanisms in food selection, the way in which such mechanisms might interact with the lifestyle changes associated with Western-style industrialisation and the implications of this for the selection of a balanced diet.

Do Humans Possess the Innate Ability to Select a Diet to Achieve Optimal Health?

In assessing the innate ability of humans to select a balanced diet (gustatory sensibility) there are two dimensions which can be considered: regulation of the intake of specific nutrients and regulation of energy intake.

Intake of Specific Nutrients

Davis [2], in a study which is frequently quoted, considered that she had found evidence for both aspects of this phenomenon. However, while this work has a certain curiosity value, the results certainly do not represent scientific evidence for gustatory sensibility because of the poor design of the study.

In an experiment which would today be considered unethical, three newly weaned infants were allowed to choose their own diet for a period of between 6 and 18 months. On the basis of her findings, Davis concluded that "they were able to select their own foods from a list of simple natural ones and in suffcent quantities to maintain themselves with apparently optimal digestive and good nutritional results. They were omnivorous and in eating were governed by their caloric needs, but showed definite preferences, which changed from time to time and were unpredictable." Davis also reported a selective preference for foods rich in vitamin D by one of the children who was suffering from active rickets when he entered the study.

Among the many criticisms which it is possible to make of the way this study was conducted and the findings interpreted, two particular problems stand out. Firstly, even though the nurses were instructed not to influence the children, it is possible that they may have done so unconsciously. Escalona [3] observed, among infants in the nursery of the Massachusetts reformatory, that babies under 4 months of age showed a consistent preference for either orange or tomato juice, which related directly to the likes and dislikes of the student nurse who cared for the infant. Changes in infant preference were seen to occur when there was a changeover in staff. This may relate also to the changes in preference observed by Davis. A second caveat relates to the nature of the foods presented to the children, which were simple and wholesome. The sweetest choices available to the children were milk and fruit, and, not surprisingly, those items were selected most often. But clearly these are foods which also provide valuable quantities of nutrients. If the study were to be repeated with items such as confectionery and fizzy drinks available, the outcome might not have been so nutritionally satisfactory.

Evidence of preferences based on needs for individual nutrients is very scanty in humans, although it has been suggested in relation to zinc deficiency [4], and as a possible explanation of pica in pregnancy. Hunter [5] suggests that minerals in clays eaten in Ghana act as dietary supplements; however, Vermeer [6,7] provides conflicting evidence concerning the calcium and magnesium content of analysed clay samples. Nonetheless it is interesting in Snow and Johnson's study [8] that some of the subjects thought that craving for starch or clay indicated a dietary need.

There is also some evidence of gustatory sensibility in relation to protein. Vazques et al. [9] demonstrated that protein-calorie malnourished children showed a preference for soup supplemented with casein hydrolysate compared with an unsupplemented soup, while Murphy [10] found that elderly subjects with a low-normal protein status (as indicated by serum albumin and blood urea nitrogen levels) displayed a preference for soups supplemented with higher levels of casein hydrolysate than did those with a better protein status.

Energy Intake

Energy intake and its regulation has received most attention because of interest in obesity and overweight. Quite large variations in body fat can be observed both between and within individuals, and it could therefore be argued that energy balance is not regulated in the same way as other parameters such as temperature. However, the precision with which any homeostatic function is regulated depends on the limits for survival, which are very narrow for temperature but considerably larger for body weight.

Since some individuals can remain for decades within 1–2 kg of their original adult weight, it has been inferred that appetite must be under remarkably good control. However such individuals may not be typical. In fact maintenance of body weight within 1–2 kg of original weight was found in less than 5% of the Framingham study population [11]. The majority did not maintain their weight so precisely but frequently displayed swings of 5–10 kg in an 18-year period of follow-up.

Nonetheless there is some evidence for the physiological regulation of food intake amongst infants and malnourished children. When the energy density of milk was manipulated [12,13] babies adjusted the quantity consumed, achieving some 80% of that required for complete compensation. Similarly, studies of small-for-dates versus large-for-dates babies [14] and of malnourished children [15] appear to demonstrate an ability to adjust intake according to physiological need.

However, it is important to remember that in these situations the effects of social pressure are at a minimum and a single food item is involved. Other studies have examined the ability of adults to adjust their food intake in response to covert alterations in the energy density of their diet. Many earlier studies involved the use of liquid diets [16–19], which are clearly an artificial situation. These studies reported varying levels of success by subjects in compensating for diluted drinks. More recently Porikos [20], in experiments with low-energy-density analogues of food in which sucrose had been replaced by aspartame, also found incomplete compensation. Similar results have been reported in other studies [21,22] using a variety of foodstuffs.

In general, results from studies in which the effect of a low or high energy pre-load on consumption of a subsequent test meal are measured have been inconclusive. Some studies [23–26] have shown clear effects of the energy content of a meal or load on later intake, while others [27–29] have failed to show any effect. One of the difficulties in drawing conclusions from studies of this kind has been the great degree of variability in the methodology adopted. The foods used differ greatly. They may be liquid, solid, or a mixture, and they may not be equally acceptable to all subjects. Furthermore, the size of the pre-load may vary from one study to another by a factor of up to 53. The nutritional composition of pre-loads may also be quite different. Quite striking differences also occur in the timing between the pre-load and the test meal or hunger rating, from only 10 minutes in one case [25] to up to 4 hours [28].

Hill et al. [30] have recently reported a study in which they attempted to deal with some of these problems of experimental methodology. After subjects had eaten either a low calorie or high calorie lunch, three measures were followed for a period of 8 hours; (1) motivational ratings, (2) preference for food items, and (3) intake from dietary records. Some evidence for incomplete compensation was produced, although the period of follow-up was considered to be a constraint.

In general, the evidence suggests that physiological adjustments do occur in response to energy intake. Under experimental conditions regulatory systems will respond to a reduction in energy intake of as little as 25% and can compensate to reduce the energy deficit to less than 15% of normal intake. However, the observed slows changes in the body weight of most adults suggest that the regulatory mechanisms controlling energy intake and expenditure are not very accurate, and can be overridden. As Table 8.1 shows, amongst the British population [31] an increasing proportion are found to be overweight or obese with increasing age.

Table 8.1. The distribution of excess weight by age in the British population, expressed in percentages

	BMI figures (inclusive)	Age (years)							All ages
		16–19	20–24	25–29	30–40	40–50	50–60	60–65	
Males									
Overweight (a)	25.0–27.9	7	17	23	28	31	32	33	27
Overweight (b)	28.0–29.9	7	2	3	5	12	11	11	7
Obese	30 and over	1	3	3	7	9	6	10	6
Total with excess weight (%)		15	22	29	40	52	49	54	39
Females									
Overweight (a)	25.0–27.9	9	15	11	15	21	25	26	18
Overweight (b)	28.0–29.9	3	3	4	6	8	9	8	6
Obese	30 and over	3	5	5	4	9	13	16	8
Total with excess weight (%)		15	23	20	25	38	47	50	32

Source: OPCS [31].

Taste as a Guide to the "Balanced Diet"

Richter [32,33] and later Rozin [34] demonstrated self-regulatory eating behaviour in rats under a number of conditions. In attempting to explain this phenomenon it has been proposed that such selection depends primarily on taste. In a series of experiments with humans, Booth [35,36] have demonstrated that adults can learn to eat smaller meals when those meals contain a disguised high calorie starch load in a soup associated with a distinctive taste.

In concentrated form starch creates a powerful but transient satiating effect after a delay following ingestion that is sufficient to allow absorption of glucose from digestion to get well under way [37]. This adaptation reported by Booth suggests that conditioned learning associated with taste occurs, and leads to an appropriate response in intake when energy density is altered by modifying starch content. The ability of protein and fat to act as conditioning agents is of considerable interest. In other experiments with rats Booth [38,39] has been able to demonstrate that disguised protein loads rapidly condition the taste preferences of hungry animals but do not condition satiety. More striking is the failure to obtain conditioning of either preferences [39] or satiation [40] by dietary fat effects. This lack of direct [24] and conditioned satiating effects of dietary fat may be particularly unfortunate in the context of any consideration of changing lifestyles and the balanced diet.

Taste has a further part to play in controlling food intake through the phenomenon described by Rolls [41–43] as "sensory-specific satiety". It is axiomatic among nutritionists that the best way to ensure nutritional adequacy is to eat a variety of foods. The work of Rolls suggests an inbuilt mechanism that helps to ensure a variety of foods is consumed. As a particular food is eaten its taste is liked less [44,42], but the taste of other foods and the desire to eat them remain relatively unchanged. Thus a desire for palatability helps to ensure selection of a varied, "nutritious" diet. The changes in liking for foods eaten and not eaten are highly correlated with the amount of those foods that will be eaten if an unexpected second course is offered [42]. This implies that more will be eaten of a varied meal than one consisting of a single food.

In a further demonstration of the effects of this phenomenon Rolls and de Waal [45] found in a long-term study that Ethiopian refugees who had been living in camps for long periods of time rated commonly provided foods as less pleasant than did the newer arrivals. The authors indicated that this could exert an impact on an individual's nutritional status, since less palatable staple foods were often traded for less wholesome items which added variety to the diet. This finding echoes the words of George Orwell in *The Road to Wigan Pier:* "When you are unemployed, which is to say you are underfed, harassed, bored and miserable, you don't want to eat dull wholesome food. You want to have something a little bit 'tasty'."

Sweet and Salt

The presence of innate preferences for sweet and salt tastes has attracted interest in considerations of the human's ability to select nutritionally optimal diets. Salt is necessary for the body to function, but is not easily available in the wild. Many species must constantly seek salt to ensure adequate intake. Therefore it would be surprising if natural selection did not favour an innate preference for salt in most species [46]. While it appears that preference for salt increases following sodium deprivation [46], other work [46a] has demonstrated that even in rats this response can be modified by social interaction. Desor et al. [47] have shown an increased preference for salty solutions in 9–15-year-old human subjects when compared with adults, and have suggested that this may be due to an increased need for sodium amongst growing subjects. However, this is consistent with the argument that preferences for salt are strongly subject to experience and learning effects, so that these findings might be explained by a cohort effect.

Similarly it has been suggested that a preference for sweet may have conferred an evolutionary advantage as it would have led animals with such a preference to an increased consumption of ripe fruits, thus boosting intake of calories, vitamins and minerals [48]. There is no doubt that genes can play a strong role in the preference for sweet in rats, and strains can be bred to have a greater or lesser preference for sweet [49]. However, this does not necessarily mean that genes make a significant contribution to the preference for sweet in humans. Although Desor et al. have documented the newborn infant's preference for sweet fluids, which suggests a strong genetic component [50], there is also some evidence for a learning effect.

Beauchamp and Moran [51] showed that among 6-month-old infants, those who were being fed sweetened water preferred it more than did others who were not being fed sweetened water.

In fact both humans and rats show a greater preference for the taste of sweet when they are young and less when they are older [47,52,53]. It has been suggested [47] that the increased caloric need of younger, pre-pubertal growing individuals automatically increases their preference for a sweet taste.

In conclusion it seems that some aspects of taste may be important in the selection of foods which are appropriate in terms of nutritional quality and quantity. Cabanac [54] has proposed the term "alliesthesia" to describe the homeostatic modulation of hedonic responses to external stimuli by internal signals. And it seems possible that hedonic conditioning may play a part in establishing preferences designed to ensure a balanced diet under circumstances where food choice is relatively limited and taste is an accurate predictor of the nutrient content of a food.

Since sensory attributes of diets from different cultures vary markedly, it has been suggested that flavour within a particular cuisine* provides important cues to ensure that foods are consumed which are safe, and provide for optimum nutrition [55–57]. These cues would have evolved on the basis of the foods that were locally available, the available technology for processing, and the nutritional value of particular food combinations. Under conditions where food availability alters and food technology permits the separation of taste from those nutrients with which the taste is naturally associated, it seems possible that the normal conditioning process designed to enhance the ability to secure a well-balanced diet may be disrupted. This will be true particularly if other environmental and social factors also have a part to play in food selection.

Both migration and industrialisation represent potentially very disruptive situations. As regards the implications of changing lifestyles for the "balanced diet" it is therefore of interest to consider whether observed changes in food habits occur in the direction which our examination of innate mechanisms would suggest, whether aspects of lifestyle act to potentiate or override these self-selection factors, and whether the results put the balanced diet at risk.

Changes in the Food Habits of Migrants: Implications for the Balanced Diet

Both humans and animals exhibit "neophobia", a fear of new things, which extends to new foods [58,59]. Studies by Pliner [60] and Birch and Marlin [61] have demonstrated that people have preferences for familiar foods. Experiments with young children have shown a clear relationship between food preference and exposure frequency. The interpretation put forward by Rozin [34] is that an organism avoids new foods because ingestion of a novel substance is risky and potentially dangerous. Successive exposures to the new substance that do not result in negative consequences reduce the negative effect, resulting in enhanced liking.

Studies which have examined changing food habits amongst immigrant groups to a number of countries have found that the amount of exposure to the host cuisine appears to be an important factor in determining the extent to which food habits alter. Bavly [62], in a study of three generations of newcomers from Europe, North Africa and the Near East to Israel, found that the extent to which food habits changed was indeed related to exposure through factors such as marriage to a member of a different ethnic group, employment of the wife outside the home, exposure to advice in the media, and indirectly through children receiving school lunches. Ability to communicate, and the degree of social interaction with the host community, seem to be important predictors of changes in food habits as indicated by several studies [63–67].

However, evidence of the effects of length of stay are conflicting. Whereas some studies [63,68] have found that longer residence is associated with greater adaptation,

*The term "cuisine" is used to characterise the food-use patterns of a particular culture and comprises four elements: (1) the foods chosen for use and criteria applied in their selection, (2) preparation methods employed, (3) characteristic flavour principles, (4) rules governing meal behaviour.

others [67,69] have found the reverse to be the case. One possible explanation is that, with a tightening of immigration regulations, younger respondents, who have been in the country for a shorter period, speak better English, are better educated and have more social contacts with the host community. A second possible explanation is that as people stay longer they discover where to purchase traditional ingredients, and so have less need to change their habits. Among several immigrant communities changes have been noted with time in the availability of traditional foods, and this has had an impact on eating habits. When numbers of immigrants were small, and perhaps involved in contract labour, they had no access to traditional foods. Once substantial numbers had arrived and diversification of employment occurred, an import–export infrastructure developed which made traditional foods available once more [70].

In any consideration of changing food habits, exposure alone clearly does not account for the adoption of some foods and not others. Any change must have more advantages than drawbacks, and it is considered that four factors impinge on the likelihood that an innovation will occur. The first is "compatibility": the extent to which the innovation is seen to be consistent with the existing needs and values of society. The second is "complexity", which relates to the degree of difficulty or effort perceived to be required in making any change. The extent to which an innovation can be experimented with on a limited basis, "trialability", will also affect the likelihood of its adoption. Such an innovation represents less risk. The final aspect, "observability", describes the degree to which the results of an innovation are obvious and the advantages consequently seen. It is interesting that whereas high fibre foods perform positively in all these areas and have found favour with consumers, advice on fat reduction is less likely to be regarded positively in respect of these factors.

Increasing consumption of dietary fibre is consistent with a popular desire to return to a simple "natural" life. It is easy to effect through a change in breakfast cereal or by adding bran to food. High fibre alternatives to familiar foods can easily be tried and the results easily observed.

In the case of immigrants, some common patterns can be seen in the adoption of new eating habits. Studies consistently show [63,65,66,68,70–72] that the most marked changes occur at breakfast, the meal with the least symbolic importance, at which convenience is a prime consideration. The shift to a Western-style breakfast based on cereals and bread or toast is widely adopted. Changes in the midday meal will depend on the extent to which the family or members of the same immigrant group eat together. But if the evening meal is the one at which most family members gather, this will be the meal which most closely resembles traditional eating patterns [62,64]. Bavly found that breakfast was taken jointly by the entire family in less than 50% of families, irrespective of generation or ethnic group, while for lunch the figures ranged from 32% to 53%. The evening meal, however, was shared by all the family members in from 48% to 92% of families, and in 70% a traditional dish would be served. This pattern illustrates both the strength of the family as a source of traditional influence tending to restrain adoption of new foods, and also the effect of changed occupational patterns which result in working mothers, fathers and children being apart on most other eating occasions.

Changes in immigrant lifestyle may place a greater emphasis on snacking or eating outside the home [64,67]. In many Western countries, those snacks most freely available and which pose no threat to traditional taboos are either savoury items of the crisp/nut variety, or sweets and confectionery, both of which we would expect to be attractive on the basis of the earlier consideration of taste. Figure 8.1 demonstrates

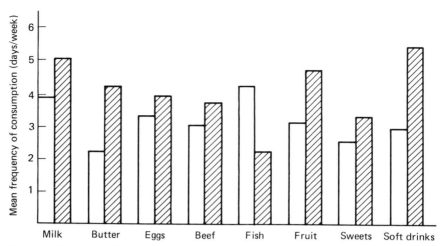

Fig. 8.1. Frequency of consumption of foods by Vietnamese in Vietnam (*open columns*) and in the United States (*hatched columns*). (From the data of Crane and Green [71].)

the changes in frequency of consumption of particular foodstuffs observed by Crane and Green [71] amongst Vietnamese living in Florida, USA. It is interesting that the pursuit of sweetness includes a significant increase in consumption of fruit, as well as soft drinks and sweets. Some foods may be incorporated into immigrant eating patterns following modification of their taste to conform to the immigrants' traditional cuisine. Thus Wenkam and Wolff [70] report Japanese immigrants in Hawaii preparing hamburger patties with Shoyu, and Rozin [56] describes the addition of soya sauce, rice wine and ginger root to create a hamburger that tastes Chinese. In this way the boundaries of what is considered to be acceptable food can be expanded.

In general it seems that changes in lifestyle lead to greater exposure to "Western foods". Within this framework a "natural tendency" to select sweet and salty foods may be reinforced by a daily pattern which encourages snacking. Exposure to a variety of new foods may encourage unnecessary energy intake. Although evidence for increasing obesity amongst immigrant groups is not available, there is considerable concern about rates of diabetes among the Asian community in the United Kingdom, which may be linked to dietary imbalances. In addition there have been reports of iron deficiency anaemia in children of immigrants to the United Kingdom due to late weaning associated with prolonged breast feeding and the late introduction of solids [73,74]. Infantile rickets continues to occur in Asian children and in a smaller proportion of West Indian children [75,76].

In consequence it would appear that the disruptions associated with migration have resulted in imbalances in the diet which self-selection mechanisms have failed to overcome.

Wenkam and Wolff [70] have attempted to compare the composition of the diets of Japanese immigrants to Hawaii over the period from the late nineteenth century to the mid 1960s, with results that indicate a steady increase in the proportion of calories from fat, as well as an increase in protein intake (Fig. 8.2). However, it is interesting that there have been changes in nutrient intakes which have taken place in Japan itself (Fig. 8.3). The similarity in trends with regard to macro-nutrient intake suggest that consumption patterns in Japan, even of traditional foodstuffs, have

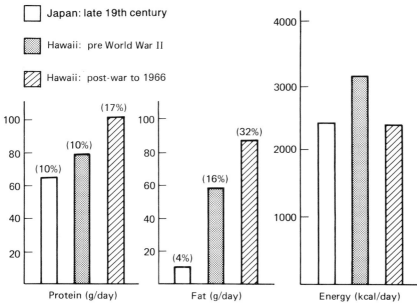

Fig. 8.2. Daily intake of protein, fat and calories among Japanese adults in Japan and Hawaii from the late nineteenth century to 1966. Figures in brackets on the tops of the columns give the percentage energy consumed as protein or fat. (After Wenkam and Wolff [70].)

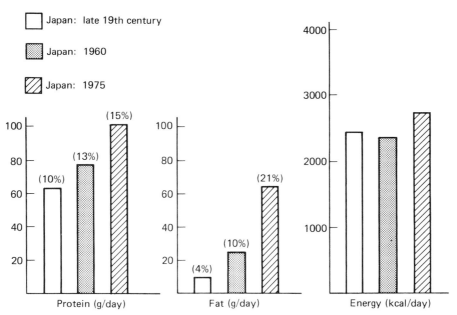

Fig. 8.3. Daily intake of protein, fat and calories amongst Japanese adults in Japan in the late nineteenth century, 1960 and 1975. Figures in brackets on the tops of the columns give the percentage of energy consumed as protein or fat. (Data from Wenkam and Wolff [70] (late nineteenth century) and Japanese National Nutritional Survey (1960 and 1975).)

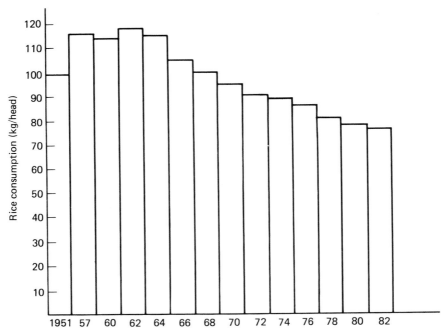

Fig. 8.4. Consumption of rice in Japan (kg/head per year).

changed. This seems to have been the case with rice (Fig. 8.4), almost certainly because of increased availability of other foods due to economic changes, differences in lifestyles and sociocultural factors. Dietary changes such as these have also been linked to conditions such as heart disease, obesity, dental disease and cancer [77–85], as discussed in other papers in this volume.

Industrialisation and Urbanisation

The changes in the nutrient composition of the diet seen amongst Japanese immigrants and in Japan itself mirror the trends which have been observed in Western Europe in the past hundred years. This period marks a critical phase in dietary change and is strongly associated with industrialisation, urbanisation and attendant changes in food availability.

Information on diets before modern times is very limited and of varying quality. Some trends, however, can be described, based principally on information concerning food availability rather than consumption. From the Middle Ages to the early modern period, virtually all of Western Europe relied on a cereal-based diet [86]. While occasional peaks of increased meat consumption occurred in periods of great demographic decline, Europe has only relatively recently moved into a situation where animal products provide more than half the dietary protein. Falls in population due to epidemics led to a restructuring of food production in the period 1300–

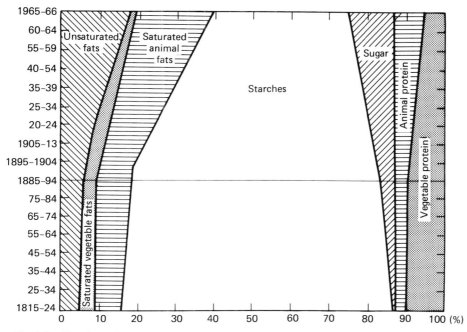

Fig. 8.5.   French nutrition 1815–1966: carbohydrates, fats and proteins. (After Toutain [87].)

1500, though it was not until the sixteenth and seventeenth centuries, with the arrival of new foods such as potatoes, maize, tomatoes, tea and coffee, that medieval diet patterns came under serious pressure. This happened first among the higher echelons of society, to be adopted later by the wider population. In the industrialised twentieth century, country after country in Europe changed from a diet dominated by cereals to one in which most of the protein was of animal origin.

In his rather speculative work, Toutain [87] has tried to trace the nutritional implications of this evolution in France, and has identified two phases. The first phase is associated with variation in quantity and regularity of calorie intake within an unchanging dietary regime; the second is characterised by an increase in fats and animal protein related to changes in the composition of the diet (Fig. 8.5). In just over 50 years France crossed the bridge which still separates the developing countries from the world's industrialised areas (Fig. 8.6).

Similar broad trends may well have occurred in Britain. As the nineteenth century progressed the pace of change in eating habits seems to have accelerated, though Dingle [89] argues that as late as the 1870s the British diet had a certain structural stability. Not before the end of the nineteenth century did a general transformation of food distribution take place. Only then did it become possible, due to an improvement in international trade and commercial channels of supply, to provide urban populations with increased quantities of meat, milk, dairy products, fresh fruits and vegetables. Tinned food became available in 1880, the year chilled meat from Australia first arrived. Within a few years pork from the United States, beef from the Argentine and lamb from New Zealand were flooding the English market. By 1902 more than 56 lb of frozen meat was consumed per head of the population per annum

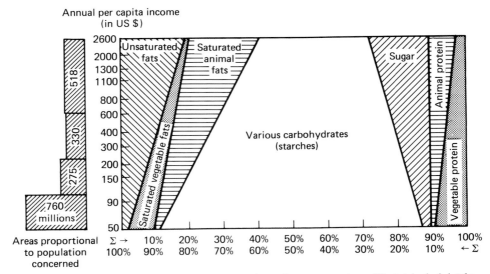

Fig. 8.6. Calories supplied by fats, carbohydrates and proteins as a percentage of the total caloric intake, by wealth of country. (After *La consommation: les perspectives nutritionelles*. Rome, 1969.)

[90]. By the early years of the twentieth century imports from the New World and Australasia had halved the cost of bread and meat to the English consumer. Consequently many families now had more income available for dairy products, fruit, vegetables and eggs, which had previously been eaten in very small quantities. In addition new products of tropical agriculture such as peanuts, bananas, pineapples and peaches arrived as quickly as conveyance by refrigerated ship or sealed can could be contrived, leading to a considerable increase in variety in the British diet.

Economics of Food Choice

As part of the process of industrialisation and urbanisation, an individual's labour became a commodity to be exchanged for cash to purchase goods and services. Clearly patterns of food consumption in an urban setting relate not only to the range of foods available, but also to the ability to purchase them. It is possible, with the greater variety of foods available, that the urban dweller may have an improved diet compared with his rural cousin. In Bangladesh, higher average consumption of meat, milk, fruit, eggs, fish, fats and oils has been reported amongst urban dwellers.

However, the distinction between socioeconomic classes may be more important in towns than rural areas. The lowest classes in slums in the peri-urban areas probably have a lower nutritional status than the poorest rural people [91]. In the cash economy, items such as housing, clothing, fuel and transport must be paid for. The proportion of income spent on food shows a consistent pattern of variation by socioeconomic group. This is clear in the cities in developing countries, and was so in Britain in the 1930s [92] and even today (see Fig. 8.7). The lowest income groups

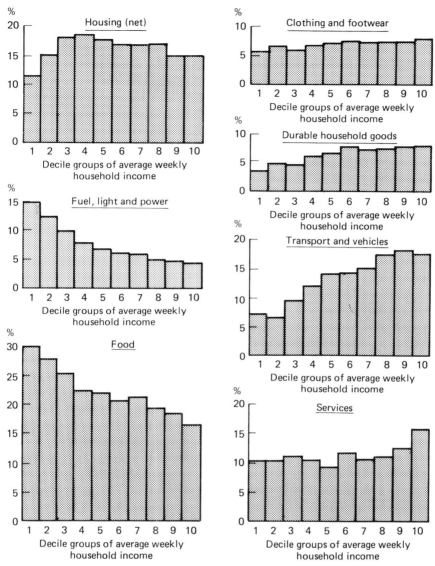

Fig. 8.7. Variation of expenditure pattern by decile group of household income, 1985. Percentages are expenditure on the commodity or service group as a percentage of total household expenditure. Income bands are decile groups of the household income distribution, group 1 being the lowest 10%. (After Family Expenditure Survey. OPCS, 1986.)

spend a higher proportion of their money on food. They buy various foods in different amounts compared with more affluent groups and may be particularly vulnerable nutritionally to changes in financial circumstances. When unexpected financial strains occur, food is the item of the budget which can most easily and quickly be modified in response [93]. Additional financial demands may tip the balance towards

Table 8.2. Mean gross weekly earnings (£) of full-time employees in Great Britain, by sex

	1970	1981	1983a	1983	1984	1985
Males						
Manual	26.2	119.0	140.1	141.6	152.7	163.6
Non-manual	34.7	159.4	190.7	191.8	209.0	225.0
All male employees	29.3	137.0	163.3	164.7	178.8	192.4
Females						
Manual	13.4	74.5	87.9	88.1	93.5	101.3
Non-manual	17.8	96.7	115.1	116.1	124.3	133.8
All female employees	16.3	91.4	108.8	109.5	117.2	126.4

Source: CSO *Social Trends* (1987).
aSeries adjusted in 1983 from a base of employees aged 18 years or over to a base of employees on adult rates.

Table 8.3. Consumers' expenditure in the United Kingdom

Percentage of total consumers' expenditure at current prices	1977	1978	1979	1980	1981	1982	1983	1984	1985 Indices/ percent- ages	£s million (current prices)
Food	18.5	17.9	17.2	16.7	15.9	15.3	15.0	14.6	14.0	29 950
Alcoholic drink	7.6	7.3	7.3	7.3	7.3	7.2	7.3	7.4	7.4	15 783
Tobacco	4.2	3.9	3.6	3.5	3.6	3.5	3.4	3.4	3.3	7 006
Clothing and footwear	7.6	7.8	7.7	7.2	6.7	6.5	6.7	6.8	7.0	14 894
Housing	13.4	13.2	13.2	13.7	14.8	15.4	15.0	14.9	14.9	31 711
Fuel and power	4.9	4.6	4.5	4.6	5.1	5.2	5.1	4.9	5.0	10 657
Household goods and services	7.3	7.6	7.6	7.3	6.9	6.7	6.7	6.6	6.6	14 067
Transport and communication	14.7	15.4	16.3	16.4	16.5	16.5	16.8	16.6	16.8	35 806
Recreation, entertainment, and education	9.3	9.4	9.3	9.3	9.2	9.2	9.1	9.2	9.2	19 593
Other goods, services,	12.6	12.9	13.3	14.1	14.0	14.4	14.9	15.6	15.8	33 741
Total	100.0	100.0	100.0	100.0	100.0	100.0	100.0	100.0	100.0	213 208

Source: United Kingdom National Accounts, Central Statistical office.

nutritional inadequacy. As McGonigle and Kirby observed, when people were moved from slums to new houses, the nutritional value of their diets was reduced [94].

What types of foods do people in low income groups in the United Kingdom say they would buy if they had more money [93]? Most frequently mentioned are meat and chicken, followed by fruit. A change which replaced the present higher consumption of meat products by meat would contribute to a reduction in the fat intake, and more fruit would improve the vitamin C intake. The "balance" of the diet would apparently improve if choice were not constrained by economic factors. It is arguable that in an urban setting, where economic factors assume greater influence on food choice, lack of money may override preferences based on gustatory sensibility.

However, in the last decade the trend in the United Kingdom has been towards higher average earnings per week (Table 8.2) and a decline in the percentage spent on food (Table 8.3). When food becomes a less important part of the budget there is more room for experimentation, so that one result of higher real incomes could be a willingness to try new foods. This could have two possible effects: it could increase variety and nutritional quality of the diet, or the taste preference for sweet and salt might lead to increased consumption of highly palatable foods of low nutrient density.

Another effect of a larger disposable income has been the increase in refrigerators, freezers and microwave ovens. Freezers are owned by three fifths of all households in the United Kingdom and might eventually reach a similar ownership level to refrigerators (over 90%). It had been thought that this would encourage storage of raw foods and home-cooked dishes; but market research has shown that most people use the freezer to store ready-meals, which may have nutritional profiles markedly different from their traditional counterparts.

Changing Roles of Women

Industrialisation has also been associated with fundamental changes in the roles of men and women. Oakley [95] suggests that the most important and enduring consequence of industrialisation for women in Britain was the emergence of the modern role of the housewife as the dominant mature female role. In the new order which followed industrialisation, work was separated from family life. While for men the range of occupations open to them expanded, the rise of housewifery as a sole occupation for married women emerged. In 1851 one in four married women (with husbands alive) was employed. By 1911 the figure was one in ten.

The nature of women's work outside the home also changed – a reflection of wider social trends. In 1851, 1881 and 1891 the majority of wage-earning women were still in the same occupations as in 1841, with domestic service and textile industries taking first and second place. Women's work in agriculture declined significantly after the late 1860s, as the need for agricultural labour generally dwindled following the invention of new machinery and the conversion of arable land to pasture. By 1900, according to the census, women's agricultural work had virtually disappeared. In 1911 more than twice as many women were employed in domestic service as in textile manufacture, and together with dressmaking these three jobs accounted for two thirds of all women's employment. But the move away from this type of work was already discernible. The number of female clerks rose from 19 in 1851 to 146 000 in 1911.

From the 1920s onwards the combined role of housewife and paid worker was a developing feature of women's situation. The percentage of the labour force made up of female workers rose from 27% in 1939 to 39% in 1945. Today [96] women form 42% of the labour force; 60% of married women under retirement age were in work in 1984, half in part-time work. Most women still have to do most of the cleaning, cooking and shopping for their families as well as going to work, so their time is under pressure. One way in which time can be saved is through the use of convenience foods. These foods may be more expensive than their equivalents produced from raw ingredients, but as the average household income rises by about £70 a week when the wife works [97], some of this extra money can be traded for convenience.

Pressure of time and a higher income militate against the use of time-consuming basic foods such as raw meat, uncooked vegetables or the production of bread and cakes at home. The demise of afternoon "tea" has also contributed to a reduction in consumption of bread and cakes, so there is no longer the same pressure on the housewife to provide these items. Separation of work and home life have had marked effects on meal patterns and the composition of meals [98].

Changes in the role of women may have a profound effect on the foods served to the rest of the family. In spite of married women's increasing employment outside the home, traditional divisions of labour within the home have proved remarkably enduring. For example, in America Walker and Woods [99] found that a husband's average time spent on all food preparation increased from 6 minutes a day when the wife was not employed to 12 minutes a day when she was. Husbands' contributions may not only be minimal, but are also usually carried out under the label of "helping out", rather than assuming responsibility for the task, and in general there is preference for rewarding rather than onerous or tedious tasks – playing with the children rather than ironing [95]. Table 8.4 indicates the division of labour in British households with regard to a number of tasks, reported in 1985 [100].

Table 8.4.   Division of labour in British households

Task	Responsibility	%
Household shopping	Mainly man	6
	Mainly women	54
	Shared equally	39
Preparation of evening meal	Mainly man	5
	Mainly women	77
	Shared equally	16
Evening washing up	Mainly man	18
	Mainly woman	37
	Shared equally	41
Household cleaning	Mainly man	3
	Mainly women	72
	Shared equally	23
Washing and ironing	Mainly man	1
	Mainly woman	88
	Shared equally	9
Repairs of household equipment	Mainly man	83
	Mainly woman	6
	Shared equally	8
Organisation of household money and bills	Mainly man	32
	Mainly woman	38
	Shared equally	28

Source: Jowell and Witherspoon [100].

Changing patterns of female employment might particularly affect the feeding of younger children, and there has been considerable interest in this as a factor affecting the decision to breast feed or bottle feed. After a steady post-war decline in breast feeding in the United Kingdom, there has been a trend in all social groups since the mid 1970s for more women to breast feed and for a longer period [101]. Surveys repeated in 1975 and 1980 showed consistently that the expectation of returning to work was not a major reason for choosing to bottle feed, being given by 6% and 5% of mothers respectively. However, international data [102] suggest that mothers who did not return to work tended to breast feed for longer than those who did go back to paid employment. Research in western Samoa [103] suggested that a key factor in the decline in the age of weaning was the increased workload for women, associated with their increasing involvement in the cash economy.

Changes in women's role may also affect the patterns of food acceptance by children. Birch [104] has discussed the transmission of stimulus control of eating behaviour, pointing out the three modes by which this may occur. Firstly, it may be a result of endogenously organised, genetically pre-programmed propensities for behaviour; secondly, similar patterns across generations may be the result of similar exposure to and experience with food due to social constraints; thirdly, transmission of behaviour can be the consequence of direct social interaction. In humans, the third form frequently involves an individual who acts as an agent of socialisation, transmitting cultural rules to the child. This is generally supposed to be principally the domain of the mother, and changes in the employment patterns of women might well affect these processes.

For example, employment might affect meal-time behaviour of mothers. Birch et al. [105] have explored mother–child interaction patterns at meal-times and their association with the degree of fatness in children. During a lunch-time situation thinner children and their mothers ate less food, at a slower rate, talked more to each other during lunch and made relatively more positive comments about the food. It is possible that working mothers may be more pressed at meal-times and tend towards the interactional characteristics associated with overweight in children, such as talking less to their children, being less responsive to their behaviour and giving the children less approval. Alternatively they might adopt the other style with a view of making meal-times an important opportunity for contact with children from whom they are separated during the working day. In a carefully executed study [106] amongst 128 pre-school children the results suggested that parental food preferences were no more strongly related to their children's preferences than are the preferences of unrelated adults of the same sub-cultural group. This suggests that it is the framework of the cuisine that may be transmitted, within which child and parent may differ in the extent to which they like or dislike individual items.

Table 8.5. Household structure in the United Kingdom (in millions)

Type of household	1961	1971	1981
Single: retired	1.19	2.20	2.77
Single: not retired	0.73	1.12	1.47
Couples	4.96	5.63	5.90
Families and children	8.22	8.14	7.71
Single parents	1.09	1.23	1.64
Total	16.19	18.32	19.49

Source: UK census figures.

In addition to changes in the role of women, other social trends have led to a larger number of households with male food preparers. This may be as a result of the increasing numbers of young people who establish single-person households (Table 8.5), or men who continue to maintain separate households following divorce (Fig. 8.8) or death of a spouse. In the United States the Census Bureau in 1981 reported 9 million non-family households headed by men, of which more than 7 million were single-person households. In addition there were nearly 2 million family households in which no wife was present.

In a study of food purchase and preparation patterns amongst this group Pearson et al. [107] found that the men studied spent a significantly larger proportion of their

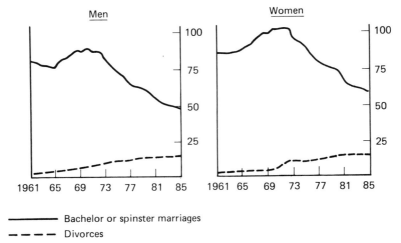

Men   Women

Fig. 8.8. Marriage and divorce rates (per 1000 eligible men or women) in Great Britain from 1961 to 1985. (Data from Office of Population Censuses and Surveys.)

food budget on complex and manufactured convenience foods. Men in the study also obtained a higher proportion of their calories from fat (41%) than did the women (34%). However, when the contribution to fat intake from convenience foods was examined, it was found to be similar in men and women (36%). In addition to concern about fat in convenience foods, there has also been concern about the contribution they may make to sodium intake. Ryley [108], in a comparison of the nutritional quality of school meals made from convenience foods compared with traditionally prepared dishes, found that convenience meals were higher in sodium than other meals. On a dry weight basis the energy density of convenience foods tended to be higher, but this was due to more carbohydrate rather than more fat.

Fast Food

Another response to the perceived lack of time for food preparation is the growth of eating outside the home and consumption of fast food in particular. Back in the 1860s, when fried fish first appeared, a piece of plaice or sole fried in batter was sold with a slice of bread for one penny and was an important addition to the often monotonous diets of ordinary working people in the cities. Today there are 11 000 or so fish and chip shops in the United Kingdom accounting for half the total fast food consumed. But now fish has been joined by pizza, hamburgers and the other items which make up the fastest-growing sector of the catering market, valued at around £1500 million a year.

There have been marked increases in the decade 1972–1982 in the consumption of takeaway food, as Table 8.6 indicates. There is also a clear trend towards the consumption of purchased meals at home, reflecting the spread of takeaways to the suburbs and the growth of video ownership. The tendency to eat fast food in the home is most marked among socioeconomic group C1 and the lower paid. The trend for "eating out at home" is regarded as a phenomenon of the 1980s, stimulated by car ownership, the trend towards more informal eating patterns, even among families, and the growth of home entertainment.

Table 8.6. Percentage of adults surveyed who claimed to have purchased takeaway food within the previous 4 weeks

Age	1972 %	1982 %
15–24	66	93
25–34	68	88
55–64	32	61

Source: Gallup Survey of Eating Out 1985.

The popularity of takeaway foods with young people (shown in Table 8.6) has led to some concerns over the nutritional implications of this trend. Nevertheless a recent survey of the dietary habits of 15–25-year-olds in the United Kingdom [109] found that in no group of subjects did the average number of takeaway meals eaten exceed one per person over a 14-day period – which would be unlikely to affect the nutritional balance of the diet.

However, an examination of the diets of British schoolchildren [110] found that boys aged 14/15 who ate their lunch at café's, fish and chip shops or takeaways (13%) had the lowest intakes of calcium, retinol equivalents, thiamin and riboflavin. Girls in this age group who followed the same lunch pattern (11%) had the lowest average daily intakes of iron, protein, calcium, nicotinic acid equivalents and vitamin D. The quality of their diets in terms of nutrients per megajoule was lower than that of any other group of girls. Younger people are more likely to miss breakfast and more likely to eat snacks [111]. As our earlier considerations on preference would suggest, these snacks may well be salty [110], or if sweet can be a major contributor to sugar intake [112].

Studies of young people [109,110] suggest that recommended intakes of nutrients are generally met, with the exception of iron. However, in the 15–25-year-old group [109] the average percentage of energy from fat consistently exceeded that recommended by the Department of Health and Social Security [113] and fibre intakes were well below that suggested by the Health Education Council [114]. Amongst the younger group [110] the fat intake of half the children fell within the range 35%–40% of total energy, while between one third and one fifth had fat intakes above 40% of energy intake, which may be considered high.

Hackett et al. [115], examining the sources of fat in adolescents' diets, found that while meat, butter or margarine and milk made the most important contributions to fat intake, confectionery, crisps, biscuits and cakes together provided over 21%. These are items which a natural preference for sweet and salty tastes would render highly palatable. It is arguable that innate preferences combine with aspects of lifestyle and available foodstuffs in such a way that certain groups in the population are at risk of dietary imbalance.

Conclusion

Food habits and food consumption patterns in Britain since World War II demonstrate the impact of many factors which have brought a demand for convenience, and a changing emphasis in meal patterns. For some groups in the population it is possible that lifestyle factors combine with innate mechanisms to influence food selection in a way which predisposes towards an "unbalanced" diet.

Table 8.7. Mean energy intake (excluding alcohol) and the fat content of the diet of the average household in Britain 1950–1986

Year	Energy (kcal)	Fat (g)	% energy from fat
1950	2470	102	36.8
1951	2470	100	36.4
1952	2450	94	34.5
1953	2520	101	36.0
1954	2630	107	36.5
1955	2640	107	36.6
1956	2620	108	37.1
1957	2590	110	38.1
1958	2600	111	38.3
1959	2580	110	38.3
1960[a]	2590	112	38.9
1960	2630	115	39.3
1961	2630	116	39.6
1962	2640	117	40.0
1963	2650	118	39.8
1964	2600	116	40.3
1965	2590	116	40.4
1966	2560	117	41.0
1967	2590	119	41.3
1968	2560	118	41.5
1969	2570	120	42.0
1970	2600	121	41.8
1971	2530	119	42.5
1972	2430	112	41.5
1973	2400	111	42.0
1974[a]	2360	110	41.9
1974	2320	106	41.3
1975	2290	107	42.2
1976	2280	105	41.7
1977	2260	105	41.9
1978	2260	106	42.0
1979	2250	106	42.4
1980	2230	106	42.6
1981	2212	103.5	42.0
1982	2172	103	43.0
1983	2144	101	42.8
1984	2063	97.2	42.8
1985	2016	95.7	42.6
1986	2064	98.1	42.6

Source: National Food Survey.
[a] Changes in survey methods resulted in two estimates.

But if we consider the overall picture, energy intakes (Table 8.7) appear to have remained quite stable between the mid 1950s and 1970s, despite growing affluence and increased variety in food availability. The increase in sugar consumption up to the mid 1960s (Table 8.8) would certainly evidence the effect of an innate preference for sweetness. This suggests that, although people have followed their natural tendency to be attracted by variety and sweetness, energy regulation mechanisms have

Table 8.8. Estimates of average household food consumption and expenditure 1950–1981

	Consumption (ounces per person per week)				
	1950	1960	1974	1981	1984
Liquid milk (pints)	4.78	4.84	4.74	4.01	3.53
Other milk (equiv. pints)	0.43	0.31	0.35	0.42	0.60
Cheese	2.54	3.04	3.74	3.89	3.60
Butter	4.56	5.68	5.61	3.69	2.87
Margarine	3.94	3.66	2.60	4.11	4.08
Lard and compound cooking fat	3.11	2.63	1.82	1.80	1.51
Eggs (number)	3.46	4.36	4.09	3.68	3.10
Preserves (incl. syrup, treacle)	6.30	3.21	2.47	2.08	1.95
Sugar	10.13	17.76	13.03	11.08	9.15
Beef and veal	8.06	8.74	7.41	6.96	6.27
Mutton and lamb	5.43	6.63	4.11	4.25	3.32
Pork	0.30	2.02	3.20	3.82	3.29
Bacon and ham (incl. cooked)	4.52	5.32	4.18	5.17	3.58
Poultry	0.35	1.68	5.18	7.30	6.97
Sausages	4.01	3.52	3.50	3.41	3.00
Other meat products	7.82	7.98	7.57	6.84	13.16
Fish, fresh and processed	6.18	4.69	2.76	2.81	1.29
Canned fish	0.44	0.95	0.60	0.69	0.70
Frozen fish and fish products	n.k.	0.29	0.96	1.42	1.56
Fresh green vegetables	13.81	15.34	12.70	11.98	10.83
Other fresh vegetables	11.38	9.13	10.20	11.83	15.26
Tomatoes, fresh	4.78	4.75	3.74	3.92	3.13
Frozen vegetables	n.k.	0.63	2.66	4.88	5.19
Canned vegetables	4.55	6.21	7.28	8.00	9.03
Potatoes (excl. processed)	62.04	56.14	45.66	38.91	39.82
Fruit, fresh	14.41	18.16	17.79	19.97	18.99
Canned fruit	3.68	6.84	4.90	2.61	2.26
Flour	7.25	6.76	5.30	5.96	4.34
White bread	50.91	36.63	28.24	21.85	20.05
Brown bread (incl. wholewheat and wholemeal)	2.55	3.35	2.64	5.56	6.51
Other bread	4.29	5.49	2.62	3.84	3.76
Buns, biscuits, cakes	10.37	11.98	10.08	9.16	8.44
Breakfast cereals	1.40	1.80	2.88	3.53	4.13
Tea	2.16	2.80	2.24	1.98	1.80
Coffee (incl. instant)	0.21	0.39	0.51	0.52	0.69
Soups	1.31	2.10	3.46	3.10	2.83

Based on data from the National Food Survey.
In 1950, rationing was still in force, though less severe than it had been. in 1960 the Macmillan government had just been re-elected on its "affluent society" platform. In 1974 recession was beginning to take effect.

operated at the same time to set limits on overall intake, against a background of declining physical effort. Since the mid 1970s average energy intake has declined, but since the beginning of the 1980s the proportions of that energy from protein, fat and carbohydrate have remained remarkably stable. It is arguable that this represents a combination of optimum palatability, and that while energy mechanisms may regulate the intake, it is affluence, food availability and taste preferences that dictate the nutrient composition. On the other hand, since foods eaten outside the home and alcohol are not reflected in the national food survey, and we know from other data that consumption of both of these have increased, it is dangerous to make inferences of this kind.

It will be interesting over the next few years to note the impact of the growing number of substitute foods with lower fat content, which allow people to enjoy the same food tastes while automatically reducing their fat and energy intake. There seems little doubt from attempts so far to monitor the impact of the "healthy eating" movement that the changes people are most prepared to make are those which require least change in terms of taste acceptability, such as using modified breakfast cereals and semi-skimmed milk.

Summary

1. There is little evidence for any innate ability to select a balanced diet. However, it is arguable that the part which taste plays in food preference may have made a contribution to the selection of a balanced diet under simple conditions, where the taste of a food was a reflection of its nutrient content.

2. Food habits have undergone various changes under the influence of industrialisation and urbanisation, with food selection influenced by increased affluence and a desire for convenience. These changes may combine with taste preferences in some groups of the population to increase consumption of certain foods at the expense of others. This leads to changes in the balance of nutrients in the diet which may have health implications, as considered in other chapters of this book.

References

1. Bingham S (1977) Dictionary of nutrition. Barrie and Jenkins, London
2. Davis CM (1928) Self selection of diet by newly weaned infants. J Dis Child 36:651–679
3. Escalona SK (1945) Feeding disturbances in very young children. Am J Orthopsychiat 15:76–80
4. Hambridge KM, Walravens PA, (1976) Zinc deficiency in infants and pre-adolescent children. In: Prasad AS (ed) Trace elements in human health and disease, vol 1. Academic Press, New York
5. Hunter JM (1973) Geophagy in Africa and the United States: A culture nutrition hypothesis. Geog Rev 63:170–195
6. Vermeer DE (1971) Geophagy among the Ewe of Ghana. Ethnology 10:56–72
7. Vermeer DE (1966) Geophagy among the Tiv of Nigeria. Assoc Am Geog Ann 56:197–204
8. Snow LF, Johnson SM (1978) Folklore, food, female reproductive cycle. Ecol Food Nutr 7:41–49
9. Vazques M, Pearson PB, Beauchamp GK (1982) Flavour preferences in malnourished Mexican infants. Physiol Behav 28:513–519
10. Murphy C (1986) The chemical senses and nutrition in the elderly. In: Kare MR, Brand JG (eds) Interaction of the chemical senses with nutrition. Academic Press, New York
11. Gordon T, Kannel WB (1973) The effects of overweight on cardiovascular disease. Geriatrics 28:80
12. Fomon SJ, Filer LJ, Thomas LN, Roger RR, Proksh AM (1969) Relationship between formula concentration and rate of growth in normal children J Nutr 198:241
13. Fomon SJ, Thomas LN, Filer LJ, Ziegler EE, Leonard MT (1971) Food consumption and growth of normal infants fed milk-based formulas. Acta Paediatr Scand [Suppl] 233
14. Ashworth A (1974) Ad Lib feeding during recovery from malnutrition. Br J Nutr 31:109
15. Ounsted M, Sleigh G (1975) The infants self-regulation of food intake and weight gain. Lancet I:1393–1397
16. Campbell RG, Hashim SA, Van Itallie TB (1971) Studies of food intake regulation in man. N Engl J Med 285:1402
17. Woolley OW (1971) Long-term food regulation in the obese and non-obese. Psychosom Med 33:436
18. Spiegel TA (1973) Caloric regulation of food intake in man. J Comp Physiol Psychol 84:24–37

19. Jordan HA (1973) Physiological control of food intake in man. In: Bray GA (ed) Obesity in perspective. Fogarty Conference, Washington, DHEW Publication NJH 75–708
20. Porikos KP (1981) Control of food intake in man: response to covert caloric dilution of a conventional and palatable diet. In: Cioffi LA, James WPT, Van Itallie TB (eds) The body weight regulatory system : normal and disturbed mechanisms. Raven Press, New York pp 83–87
21. Stockley L, Jones FA, Broadhurst AJ (1984) The effects of moderate protein or energy supplements on subsequent nutrient intake in man. Appetite 5:209–219
22. Durrant ML, Royston JP, Wloch RT, Garrow JS (1982) The effect of covert changes in energy density of pre-loads on subsequent adlibitum energy intake in lean and obese human subjects. Hum Nut Clin Nut 36C:297–306
23. Pliner P (1973) Effect on liquid and solid pre-loads on eating behaviour of obese and normal persons. Physiol Behav 11:285–90
24. Geliebter AA (1979) Effects of equicaloric loads of protein, fat and carbohydrate on food intake in the rat and man. Physiol Behav 22:267–273
25. Kissileff HR, Gruss LP, Thornton J, Jordan HA (1984) The satiating effects of foods. Physiol Behav 32:319–332
26. Birch LL, Deysher M (1985) Conditioned and unconditioned caloric compensation: evidence for self-regulation of food intake in young children. Learn Motiv 16:341–355
27. Woolley SC (1972) Physiological versus cognitive factors in short term regulation in the obese and non-obese. Psychosom Med 34:62–68
28. Speigel TA (1973) Caloric regulation of food intake in man. J Comp Physiol Psychol 84:24–37
29. Rolls BJ, Hetherington M, Burley VJ, Van Duijenvoorde PM (1986) Changing hedonic responses to foods during and after a meal. In: Kare MR, Brand JG (eds) Interaction of the chemical senses with nutrition. Academic Press, New York
30. Hill AJ, Leathwood PD, Blundell JE (1987) Some evidence for short-term caloric compensation in normal weight human subjects: the effects of high and low energy meals on hunger, food preferences and food intake. Hum Nut Appl Nutr 41A:244–257
31. Office of Population Censuses and Surveys (1981) OPCS Monitor, ref SS 81/1
32. Richter CP (1942) Self selection of diets. J Pediatr 20:230–236
33. Richter CP (1947) Biology of drives. J Comp Physiol Psychol 40:129–134
34. Rozin P (1976) The selection of foods by rats, humans and other animals. In: Rosenblatt JS et al. (eds) Advances in the study of behaviour, vol 6. Academic Press, New York
35. Booth DA, Lee M, McAleavey C (1976) Acquired sensory control of satiation in man. Br J Psychol 67:137–147
36. Booth DA (1981) Hunger and satiety as conditioned reflexes. In: Weiner H, Hofer MA, Stunkard AJ (eds) Brain behaviour and bodily diseases. Raven Press, New York
37. Booth DA (1979) Metabolism and the control of feeding in man and animals. In: Brown K, Cooper SJ (eds) Chemical influences of behaviour. Academic Press, New York
38. Booth DA (1974) Acquired sensory preferences for protein in diabetic and normal rates. Physiol Psychol 2:344–348
39. Booth DA, Stoloff R, Nicholls J (1974) Dietary flavour acceptance in infant rats established by association with effects of nutrient composition. Physiol Psychol 2:313–319
40. Booth DA (1972) Conditioned satiety in the rat J Comp Physiol Psychol 81:457–471
41. Rolls BJ, Roe EA, Rolls ET, Kingston B, Megson A, Gunary R (1981) Variety in a meal enhances food intake in man. Physiol Behav 26:215–221
42. Rolls BJ, Rolls ET, Rowe EA, Sweeney K (1981) Sensory specific satiety in man. Physiol Behav 27:137–142
43. Rolls BJ, Van Duijenvoorde PM, Rolls ET (1984) Pleasantness changes and food intake in a varied four course meal. Appetite 5:337–348
44. Rolls BJ, Rowe EA, Rolls ET (1980) Appetite and obesity: influences of sensory stimuli and external cues. In: Turner MR (ed) Nutrition and lifestyles. Applied Science Publishers, London
45. Rolls ET, de Waal AWL (1985) Long-term sensory specific satiety: evidence from an Ethiopian refugee camp. Physiol Behav 34:1017–1020
46. Denton D (1982) The hunger for salt. Springer-Verlag, Berlin Heidelberg New York
46a. Galef BG (1986) Social interaction modifies learned aversions, sodium appetite and both palatability and handling time-induced preferences in rats. J Comp Psychol 100:432–439
47. Desor JA, Greene LS, Maller O (1975) Preferences for sweet and salty in 9–15 year old and adult humans. Science 190:686–687
48. Rozin P (1976) The selection of foods by rats, humans and other animals. In: Rosenblatt JS et al. (eds) Advances in the study of behaviour, vol 6. Academic Press, New York
49. Nachman M (1959) The inheritance of saccharin preference. J Comp Physiol Psychol 52:451–457

50. Desor JA, Maller O. Turner RE (1973) Taste in acceptance of sugars by human infants. J Comp Physiol Psychol 84:496–501
51. Beauchamp GK, Moran M (1982) Dietary experience and sweet taste preference in human infants. Appetite 3:139–152
52. Wurtman JJ, Wurtman RJ (1979) Sucrose consumption early in life fails to modify the appetite of adult rats for sweet foods, Science 205:321–322
53. Logue AW, Smith ME (1986) Predictors of food preferences in humans. In: Logue AW (ed) The psychology of eating and drinking. WH Freeman, New York
54. Cabanac M (1971) Physiological role of pleasure. Science 173:1103–1107
55. Lee D (1957) Cultural factors in dietary choice. Am J Clin Nutr 5:166–170
56. Rozin P (1978) The use of characteristic flavourings in human culinary practice. In: Apt CM (ed) Flavour: its chemical, behavioural and commercial aspects. Westview Press, Colorado
57. Rozin E (1982) The structure of cuisine. In: Barker LM (ed) The psychobiology of human food selection. AVI Publishing, Westport
58. Hill WF (1978) Effects of mere exposure on preferences in non-human animals. Psychol Bull 85:1177–98
59. Zajonc RB (1968) Attitudinal effects of mere exposure. J Pers Soc Psychol [Monograph Suppl 9] (2):1–27
60. Pliner P (1982) The effects of mere exposure on liking for edible substances. Appetite 2:283–290
61. Birch LL, Marlin DW (1982) I don't like it. I never tried it. Effects of exposure on two year old children's food preferences. Appetite 3:353–360
62. Bavly S (1966) Changes in food habits in Israel. J Am Diet Assoc 48:488–495
63. Ho GP, Nolan FL, Dodds ML (1966) Adaptation to American dietary patterns by students from oriental countries. J Am Diet Assoc 58:277–280
64. Hunt S (1977) Adaptation and nutritional implications of food habits among Ugandan Asians settling to Britain. Ph.D. thesis, London Unversity
65. Krondl M, Hrboticky N, Coleman P (1984) Adapting to cultural changes in food habits. In: White PL, Selvey N (eds) Malnutrition: determinants and consequences. Alan R Liss, New York
66. Grivetti LE, Paquette MB (1978) Non traditional ethnic food choices among first generation Chinese in California. J Nutr Educ 10:109–112
67. Hsia PYK, Yeung DL (1976) A dietary study of adult Chinese Canadians in Vancouver. J Can Diet Assoc 37:164–173
68. Yang G, Fox HM (1979) Food habit changes of Chinese persons living in Lincoln, Nebraska. J Am Diet Assoc 75:420–424
69. Al Mokhalalati J (1981) A study of changing food habits among Sudanese students in Britain. Ph. D. thesis, London University
70. Wenkam NS, Wolff RJ (1970) A half century of changing food habits among Japanese in Hawaii. J Am Diet Assoc 57:29–32
71 Crane NT, Green NR (1980) Food habits and food preferences of Vietnamese refugees in North Florida. J Am Diet Assoc 76:591–593
72. Lewis JS, Ita CJ (1980) Food habits and nutrient intakes of Korean women who have migrated from Korea to Los Angeles. Fed Proc 39:653
73. Hunt SP, O'Riordan JLH, Windo J, Truswell AS (1976) Vitamin D status in different subgroups of British Asians. Br Med J ii:1351
74. Stroud CE (1971) Nutrition and the immigrant. Br J Hosp Med 5:629–634
75. Gertner JM, Lawrie B (1977) Preventing nutritional rickets. Lancet I:257
76. Dunnigan MG, McIntosh WB, Sutherland et al. (1981) Policy for prevention of Asian rickets in Britain. A preliminary assessment of the Glasgow rickets campaign Br Med J 282:357–360
77. Marmot MG, Syme SL, Kagan H, Cohen J, Belsky J (1975) Epidemiologic studies of coronary heart disease and stroke in Japanese men living in Japan, Hawaii and California. Am J Epidemiol 106:514
78. Yano K, Blackwelder WC, Kagan A, Rhoadds GG, Cohen JN, Marmot MG (1979) Childhood cultural experience and the incidence of CHD in Hawaiian Japanese men. Am J Epidemiol 109:440
79. Hankin J, Reed D, Labarthe D, Nichaman M, Stallones R (1970) Dietary and disease patterns among Micronesians. Am J Clin Nutr 23:346–357
80. Calloway DH, Gibbs JC (1976) Food patterns and food assistance programs in Cocopah Indian Community. Ecol Food Nutr 5:183–196
81. Haenszel W, Kuritan M (1968) Studies of Japanese migrants. Mortality from cancer and other diseases amongst Japanese in the United States. J Natl Cancer Inst 40:43–68
82. Muto S (1977) Dietary Sweet. Exposure and preference among Japanese children and in laboratory rats. In: Taste and development: the genesis of sweet preference. DHEW, Bethesda

83. Toshio O (1978) Anthropometric and disease pattern changes in the Japanese population: nutritional or other? In: Margen S, Ogar RA (eds) Progess in human nutrition. AVI Publishing, Westport
84. Draper HH (1977) The Aboriginal diet in modern perspective. Anthropologist 79:309–316
85. Schaeffer O, Temmermans JFW, Matthews AR (1980) General and nutritional health in two Eskimo populations at different stages of acculturation. Can J Publ Health 71:397–405
86. Aymard M (1979) Towards the history of nutrition: some methodological remarks. In: Forster R, Ranum O (eds) Food and Drink in History. Johns Hopkins University Press, Baltimore
87. Toutain JC (1971) La consommation alimentaire en France de 1789 à 1964. Economies et Societas, Cahiers de l'ISEA, Geneva
88. FAO (1969) La consommation, les perspectives nutritionelles et les politiques alimentaires. In: Plan indicatif mondial provisoire pour le developpement de l'agriculture, vol 2, chapt 13. FAO, Rome
89. Dingle RE (1972) Drink and working class living standards in Britain 1870–1914. Econ Hist Rev 608–622
90. Burnett J (1979) Plenty and want. A social history of diet in England from 1815 to the present day. Scolar Press, London
91. FAO/WHO (1971) Food and nutrition in urban slums and shanty towns. Paper presented to UNICEF, Geneva, 1971. FAO, Rome
92. Boyd Orr J (1936) Food, health and income. Macmillan, London
93. McKenzie JC (1980) Economic influences on food choice. In: Turner M (ed) Nutrition and lifestyles. Applied Science Publishers, London
94. McGonigle GCM, Kirby J (1936) Poverty and public health. Victor Gollancz, London
95. Oakley A (1976) Housewife. Allen Lane, London
96. CSO (1987) Social trends 17. HMSO, London
97. OPCS (1986) Family expenditure survey. HMSO, London
98. Thomas JE (1982) Food habits of the majority : evolution of the current UK pattern. Proc Nutr Soc 41:211–227
99. Walker K, Woods ME (1976) Time use: a measure of household production of family goods and services. American Home Economics Association Centre for the Family, Washington D.C.
100. Jowell R, Witherspoon S (1985) British social attitudes. Gower, London
101. Martin J, Monk J (1982) Infant feeding 1980. OPCS/HMSO, London
102. WHO (1981) Contemporary patterns of breast-feeding. WHO, Geneva
103. Nardi BA (1984) Infant feeding and women's work in Western Samoa. Ecol Food Nutr 4:277–286
104. Birch LL (1987) The acquisition of food acceptance patterns in children. In: Bookes RA, Popplwell DA, Burton MJ (eds) Eating habits: food physiology and learned behaviour. John Wiley, Chichester
105. Birch LL, Marlin DW, Kramer L, Peyer C (1981) Mother–child interaction patterns and the degree of fatness in children. J Nut Educ 13:17–21
106. Birch LL (1980) The relationship between childrens food preferences and those of their parents. J Nutr Educ 12:14–18
107. Pearson JM, Capps O, Axelson J (1986) Convenience food use in households with male food preparers. J Am Diet Assoc 86:339–334
108. Ryley, J (1984) The nutritional quality of school meals made from convenience foods compared with traditionally prepared dishes. Hum Nutr Appl Nut 38A:42–49
109. Bull N (1985) Dietary habits of 15–25-year-olds. Hum Nutr Appl Nutr 39: [suppl]1–68
110. Wenlock RW, Disselduff MM, Skinner RK, Knight I (1986) The diets of British schoolchildren. DHSS/OPCS, London
111. Health Promotion Research Trust (1987) The health and lifestyle survey. HPRT, London
112. Rugg-Gunn DR, Hackett AF, Appleton DR, Moynihan PJ (1986) The dietary intake of added and natural sugars in 405 English adolescents. Hum Nutr Appl Nutr 40A:115–124
113. DHSS (1984) Diet and cardiovascular disease. Committee on medical aspects of food policy: report of the panel on diet in relation to cardiovascular disease. Report on health and social subjects 28. DHSS, London
114. NACNE (1983) Proposals for nutritional guidelines for health education in Britain. Health Education Council, London
115. Hackett AF, Rugg-Gunn AJ, Appleton DR, Coombs A (1986) Dietary sources of energy, protein, fat and fibre in 375 English adolescents. Hum Nutr Appl Nutr 40A:176–184

Commentary

Southgate: The preference for sweet taste does appear to be innate but it could be argued that it is a protection against consuming bitter plant foods. It is extremely difficult to argue that this preference ensures adequate energy intake, since most energy-rich foods are not sweet.

An understanding of the factors affecting food choice is clearly crucial to the development of rational approaches to dietary change. Thomas's paper illustrates the complexity of the issues involved and alludes to the experimental difficulties in this field of research. This extensive review provides a good coverage of the evidence relating to gustatory effects on food choice. The evidence that these in themselves are adequate to ensure a balanced diet in an environment when other pressures for dietary change abound is not convincing, unless the incidence of diseases with a supposed dietary component is related to changes within the compositional domains presently regarded as balanced.

Chapter 9

Towards a National Food and Nutrition Policy

J. P. W. Rivers

Introduction

The proposal that the United Kingdom needs a national food and nutrition policy is one which commands considerable public and press support (see, for example, Cannon [9]). The debate on this need has tended to be treated as purely a matter of public health policy, with the quality of the evidence for diet/disease relationships being the only touchstone for making a decision. The nature of these relationships, and the quality of the scientific evidence pertaining to them, has been discussed by the other authors in this book. There is no need to reiterate them here. Instead I shall confine myself to exploring more generally some of the other issues involved in moving from nutrition science to policy.

Humpty Dumpty's dictum that "words mean what I want them to mean, neither more nor less" is a useful one in such a discussion, so I shall begin by defining what I understand "food policy" and "nutrition policy" to be.

As I interpret it, food policy is something developed by the State and operating at the national level. Food policy modifies patterns of production, supply, manufacture or purchasing of foods, by a mixture of legal controls and fiscal incentives or disincentives. Food policy can have a variety of objectives.

Nutrition policy, on the other hand, is the attempt to modify consumption for health reasons. Nutrition policy can be incorporated into food policy, thus providing one of its objectives. Alternatively the goals of nutrition policy can be achieved by less interventionist means, primarily by publicising guidelines to inform consumers, institutional caterers or even the food industry, or for use in education.

In my view there is no question as to whether we need national food or nutrition policies; we already have them. The State has convened committees to examine nutrition policy for more than 50 years [12], while food policy has a much longer history, the State having considered, and intermittently applied food policies in this country for at least the 700 years since the Assize of Bread in 1266 first regulated the price and size of loaves of brown and white bread. Therefore the only debate which we can still have is what such policies should be today and how they should be developed. The former is what scientists tend to concentrate upon. I shall pay attention to the latter, which I believe must be resolved before the nature of the policy can even be considered.

It is a truism that policy is devised by the State; the role of scientists is merely to advise. Unfortunately in such areas the State is a Black Box, and just how it develops policy is mysterious. All we have to guide us in considering it are *post hoc* models devised by academics from the various actions of the State, on the assumption that there is in fact some underlying coherence in the process of decision-making [1,2].

Though governments may in fact work by muddling through, a process dignified academically as incrementalism [3], we must hope that this takes place within an ideal of strategic planning whereby policy is developed by the rational consideration of policy alternatives with their costs and benefits. Of course, imperfect perception of these may require frequent changes of direction, but that need not negate the reality of an attempt to steer the ship of State.

In this discussion I assume that such a dedication to strategy exists even if it is submerged beneath the muddle. The debate, therefore, is about what steps should be taken to make such policies internally consistent in the way in which they deal with the various issues upon which a food policy impinges, and in particular how conflicts in outcomes should be resolved.

To many in the health sciences the debate is a simple one, since there is no conflict between differing outcomes of policy. According to this view it is self-evident that food policy should be subservient to nutrition policy, that is designed to maximise the health of the consumer. However noble and desirable such an end may be to us, we may be assured that the State does not see it in this way. Nor should it. Quite what the State does exist to do has been addressed by political theorists from Machiavelli onwards, and it hardly becomes me to attempt to contribute to such a distinguished debate. But it is clear that the State does not exist simply to maximise the health of its component members. Otherwise in most circumstances no State would have ever declared war, a process which, whatever the political gains, costs lives.

Costs and Benefits in Framing Policy

Evidently, therefore, the State develops many policies according to criteria which, while they might include health, are not solely dedicated to it. Policy will be decided by resolving which criteria should be included as its objectives and what weighting should be given to them.

The question of weighting is of vital importance in this, as in so many policy areas, because the costs and benefits of a policy are dissimilar in kind. If policy is to be developed rationally, therefore, costs and benefits have to be weighted so as to convert them into a common currency in which they may be compared. Yet this process, which is at the centre of policy frameworks, is intrinsically subjective and non-scientific.

The problem can be illustrated by an example far from the food and health arena: that of nuclear weapons policy. The arguments for and against unilateral nuclear disarmament could be expressed as:

1. Our possession of nuclear weapons has reduced the possibility of war in Europe and therefore has occasioned considerable savings of life, property and environment.

2. Our possession of nuclear weapons makes a war, should it occur, likely to be far more destructive in terms of its impact on life, property and environment.

3. Our nuclear weapons carry with them a clear possibility of an accident, which would cause extensive damage to life, property and environment.

If those were the sole arguments in favour of or against nuclear weapons, a rational policy of retention or abolition could in theory be developed. Since all the outcomes are similar in kind, by assigning numerical values to the various probabilities listed, an objectively "best" policy could be devised.

But once other factors are introduced, such as that Britain should retain its nuclear weapons to keep a seat at the "Top Table", or that Britain should renounce such weapons because they are immoral, no objective resolution of the argument is possible. Though we may not express it in these terms, nor even consciously make the equation, we are introducing quite arbitrary weighting factors such as the number of man-years of life placed at risk which are equivalent to a seat at the "Top Table", or the number of man-years of life we would place at risk for the right to uphold our personal idea of morality.

There seems to me to be one other aspect of the nuclear weapons debate that is pertinent to a debate about food policy and health. To appear to set human life against other avowed objectives is of course so unacceptable, not merely politically but to the overall sense of moral values in our society, that this equation is not overtly made. No one wants to admit to undervaluing human life. Therefore nuclear weapons debates tend to take place with each side arguing about the risks such weapons carry. This is a curiosity, since given adequate research, those risks can be more or less objectively assessed. But then both sides in the debate would be politically naked, forced to make it clear at what value in human lives each side set their moral and political objectives. Rather than try to persuade the public that this is an acceptable price, it is easier to argue about the validity of the research.

This analysis is a superficial one but I hope it serves to illustrate the limits of objectivity in policy that heterogeneity of costs and benefits in outcome imposes. Food and nutrition policy is no less subject to such constraints than purely "political" policy issues, and these constraints cannot be unequivocally resolved.

Examples of the costs of food and nutrition policy are fairly obvious. There is a tendency amongst diet reformers to see them always in terms of food industry profits, and hence to argue the paranoid case that government inaction is always due to a mysterious wish to protect the industry. This may be so, but, as far as I can see, much of the traditional food industry is making more, not less, profit out of the new wish for "healthy" diets, and a bevy of smaller "health food companies" seem to be developing in its wake. The costs of policy are much more widespread than these, however.

As Payne and I have argued elsewhere [4], there are costs arising from the fact that food policies will almost certainly have different impacts on different sections of the population. Policies which provide an effective disincentive to, for example, salt consumption will have an impact in terms of reduced freedom of choice on the whole population, yet their benefits are likely to be preferentially felt by only a small section of that population who are at high risk of disease.

Payne and I argued that it is both the variability of intake and the disease risk/intake curve that determine the extent of this inequity, and that without information on these two parameters policy choices will be fundamentally flawed.

As such information is obtained, the disparity between individual costs and benefits can be improved by targeting, aimed specifically at modifying the consumption patterns of high-risk subgroups. Consider, for example, Rose's example of the reduction in blood pressure by 2 mmHg discussed by MacGregor (Chap. 5) and by Sanders in the accompanying Commentary. MacGregor argues that a reduction in salt intake is a good method of achieving a fall in blood pressure, and that a linear relationship exists between blood pressure and salt intake. To achieve Rose's target, therefore, everyone must reduce salt intake by the same amount.

For individuals with a low salt intake this involves the biggest proportional reduction in intake, and hence the most noticeable change in their diet. Yet each of these generally normotensive individuals will reap the smallest health benefit. By contrast, targeting the advice at high salt consumers will, assuming the correctness of MacGregor's hypothesis, ensure that individuals will receive the greatest benefit per unit of "dietary effort", and that the smallest possible group make changes from which they are unlikely to benefit.

Of course such targeting is not necessarily in the State's interest. As MacGregor argues, the maximum impact on the health of the nation, and hence the maximum health-care saving, will be made if everyone modifies their diet. Resolving this conflict between individual choice and collective responsibility [20] is one of the political problems that suffuse this debate.

Other examples of nutritional targetting would be advice to reduce dietary fat to 35% of energy intake, which, Southgate pointed out, is a self-targeting strategy which does not constrain consumers of more prudent diets. Targeting dietary measures towards specific physiological or social groups, such as UK Asians, who are in some way at high risk, would also improve the cost–benefit ratio.

Nevertheless public health measures will always involve a price paid by the many for benefit felt by the few. As a scientist I see no objective way of justifying this, though as a political animal I am quite content that this should occur. Scientific research will not resolve this dilemma, though as explained it might do much to alter the political acceptability or unacceptability of any strategies.

Many other costs may exist besides dietary constraints. It may be the case that different food policies have different outcomes in terms of mortality and morbidity or even in terms of morbidity from different causes; there are no objective weightings possible there. Another example might be that a food policy will improve health, but that the changes in agricultural practice which would follow would increase rural unemployment and lead to changes in the amenity value of the countryside.

Of course the more policy is targeted, the less its peripheral impact will be. If a small group of individuals changes its behaviour, there will still be some impact on society in general, though there will obviously be less "fallout" the fewer people who change. I do not think that targeting is without problems. It is difficult to fit within a national food policy, though it is easier to do so if the objective is to increase consumption of certain foods amongst the poor, rather than to reduce it amongst the more affluent. In many cases, therefore, it is part of a nutrition policy, only aimed at informing so as to change behaviour. Such programmes inevitably spill over, modifying the behaviour of non-risk groups. Finally, targeting can be expensive if the high-risk groups are not self-selecting and less than obvious; if, for example, they are, as Naismith has suggested, genetically vulnerable.

Notwithstanding all this, it seems to be that in general the gain of improved health for some must be weighed against a loss of quality of life for others. I cannot conceive of a process whereby outcomes as different as the quality of life for some and mortality risk for others can be objectively equated. Such problems exist and mean that decisions about food policy will always ultimately be non-scientific, whatever we pretend to the contrary.

In my experience such arguments are not considered enough by commentators in the food and nutrition field. Indeed, when they are advanced they tend to get dismissed: how can a trivial loss of freedom be compared to the loss of a single human life? Yet the State tolerates a considerable mortality on the roads so that some may have the freedom to drive, and a massive mortality from alcohol-related causes so that some may drink. This is no different to not taxing fat, at a cost of heart disease deaths.

These are tacit cost–benefit decisions; overt ones have a considerable currency in health planning, and cost–benefit analysis is now a standard way of discriminating between treatments in the National Health Service, where, since outcomes are essentially similar, it is a fairly easy process to apply [5]. It is also applied in some areas of social policy planning; for example siting of traffic lights, where reduced accident risk is weighed against impact on traffic flow, with an arbitrary value being assigned to human life. Someone somewhere in the government machine must be applying them to nutrition, even if imperfectly and casually. I only hope they bear in mind Lord Rothschild's maxim: "I sometimes think that when talking or reading about risk, the most dangerous word in the English Language is 'professor'" [6].

Costs and Benefits in Policy and Structure of Decision-Making in Science

It is not for the scientific adviser to weigh all the diverse outcomes that may flow from policy. But equally one cannot simply argue that since the scientists' job is to provide the scientific grist for the decision-makers' mill, policy is not the concern of scientists, since the non-health aspects of the food policy nexus impinge on the decision-making process scientists employ.

This interaction comes at the level of the degree of proof that scientists require to accept the medical implications of food policy. If there were no non-health aspects to any policy, a committee would only have to weigh up the evidence of health benefit against that of direct harm to decide which was the better course of action. Yet advisory bodies such as the Committee on Medical Aspects of Food Policy (COMA) do not always do this. Rather they sometimes produce conclusions of the form that while there is some evidence for benefit, this evidence falls short of proof, and therefore apparently is not yet sufficient to justify action. Thus COMA wrote in 1974:

The Panel unanimously agreed that they cannot recommend an increase in the intake of polyunsaturated fatty acids in the diet as a measure intended to reduce the risk of ischaemic heart disease. In their opinion the available evidence that such a dietary alteration would reduce that risk in the United Kingdom is not convincing. [7]

In making such statements, COMA either assumed that the criteria of proof in formulating policy should be the same as those internal to science, or implicitly accepted that action has some disadvantage or cost outside the sphere of health.

For diet/health relationships to be judged by stringent conventional scientific criteria when formulating policy is to place this part of the policy framework at a selective disadvantage to the rest, which uses much softer criteria. Moreover strict scientific proof is unnecessary if arbitrary cost–benefit criteria will be applied to a putative diet/health relationship in policy synthesis. It is appropriate to ask, therefore, whether strict scientific criteria of proof that a relationship exists between diet and disease, should be modified in public health work.

For me this issue was brought into sharp focus by the decision in October 1985 by the US National Academy of Sciences (NAS) not to release the official report on Recommended Daily Allowances (RDAs) that an expert committee had spent 5 years compiling [21,22]. The committee's report was apparently unacceptable because it reduced the RDAs for vitamins A and C, at a time when many diet health activists wanted them increased, and when poverty campaigners felt that this decision would lead to a decline in the quality of school lunch programmes and reductions in the food stamp systems [21,22].

They may have been right, but as Kamin, the chairman of the committee argued: "Shall scientific committees give the best advice they can, or that which pleases a generation of policy makers, [and should] science be a slave of policy?" [cited in 21].

In his inaugural lecture as Professor of Community Medicine at University College London, Marmot summed up the problem:

This lust for absolute "proof" represents a view of science that is mistaken, dangerously so, since it interferes with two types of endeavour: translating scientific evidence into public health policy and pursuing research into the social causation of disease. [8]

I write this paper as someone who, as a scientist, is still unconvinced by many current hypotheses about diet and degenerative disease. But I must admit that the consensus as it currently exists, and the quality of the evidence, while it falls far short of scientific proof, exceeds the level of proof employed in more purely political spheres.

It would be premature to conclude that scientists should simply relax their burden of proof in diet/health issues. Yet when a science is incorporated into public policy, there is a need to reassess the role of proof within the structure of that science.

As well as Marmot, another person who has addressed these problems specifically with regard to food policy is Cannon in his book *The Politics of Food* [9]. Cannon unfortunately buries his discussion deep in an overly long book the tenor of which almost guarantees that he will not be taken seriously be scientists or politicians. However, what he has to say is to the point:

All expert committees concerned with food and public health both in Britain and other countries and those that advise international agencies such as the World Health Organisation are judicial: they are, in effect, tribunals, and are established to hear evidence and make judgements . . . It follows that the job of such expert committees is to produce a verdict based either on the standard of proof required in a civil court (balance of probability) or else in a criminal court (beyond reasonable doubt); and that proof in this context cannot be defined in any other way. That is to say, there is of course scientific evidence concerning food and public health, but there is no such thing as "scientific proof". It is a meaningless phrase unless it means "a judgement based on scientific evidence". [9]

Cannon's analysis does not go far enough, and raises as many questions as it resolves. "Beyond reasonable doubt" would, for example, be a difficult concept to apply unless one decided whether theories of disease were to be regarded as provisionally true until proven false, as Popper [10] argues that scientists should; or false until proven true, which Popper [10] tells us is impossible, but which most administrators would prefer since it creates stability in policy. It leaves unresolved the practical issues of who would convene these scientific tribunals, how the procedure of appointment to them should proceed, and how they would decide whether the evidence was adequate. Moreover Cannon [9] blurs the distinction between a committee which exists within the structure of government to help make policy, and one which exists outside it to exert political pressure on policy-makers. These two must be considered separately.

Experts and Committees: Scientists and Pressure Groups

Various aspects of this are important. One of these is the actions of those of us who are "cynics", and who may find ourselves therefore requested to speak or write by public relations consultants briefed by the food industry to defend a food that is under attack. In a scientific debate such devil's advocacy is a good thing since it serves to prevent a consensus being established by the winds of fashion which blow through science as through other fields of human endeavour. But in extreme cases it gets difficult to defend. Moreover where such PR output is intended for the press, or directly aimed at the public, it is difficult to see this as part of a scientific debate. Cannon [9] lists some examples of this phenomenon, and it is one which, in my experience, causes much outrage; but short of imposing professional constraints of a sort that would be unacceptable to most scientists I think it is something we just have to live with.

Equally it is difficult to justify the extent to which the advocates of comprehensive changes in our diet have used a largely non-governmental expert committee structure to impose their view on government, the scientific community and the public. While the official UK government Committee on Medical Aspects of Food Policy (COMA) dithered indecisively in the 1970s, a host of unofficial reports on diet and health, of which NACNE [11] was the most famous, were used very effectively to create a feeling of consensus in the scientific community about this issue.

Yet the process was more than a little suspect. Quite why sponsoring bodies such as the Royal College of Physicians, the British Nutrition Foundation or the Health Education Council felt they needed to produce such reports I do not know, but their backing was crucial to the effectiveness of the reports. The grand imprimatur of the sponsors served to obscure the fact that the views were those of a small group of scientists who happened to sit on the committees. Moreover the different sponsorships hid the fact that these reports were not independent since there was considerable overlap in the membership of the committees.

In many ways the process was a repetition of that which occurred in the 1930s when a coalition of nutritionists and public health reformers set up the Campaign against Malnutrition, to force the hand of a government they felt was insufficiently concerned about food and health. This campaign served amongst other things to increase the hold of the vitamin lobby, who held that poor diets were a cause of much ill health and underperformance, and further to weaken already beleaguered dissenting scientists such as Professor Cathcart, who did not see subclinical vitamin deficiency as so important and held that overall food intake, constrained by poverty, was a factor to be considered [12].

More recently the 1973 WHO/FAO report of the Expert Committee on Energy and Protein Requirements [13] was challenged by semi-official alternative committees such as the UNU one which sought to campaign against its report.

In one sense, these quasi-official expert committees are of course part of the way in which a pluralist democracy, like ours, functions: they are one of the pressure groups whereby the citizen amplifies his voice [2,3]. But they are more than this, since both their assumption of a cloak of scientific prestige from the sponsoring agency, and the fact that the logic of their considerations is opaque to all but a few scientists, means that their function is not to contribute to an informed debate but to bludgeon into silence by the invocation of expertise. Scientific pressure groups are of a special kind, uniquely powerful; evidence indeed that science is the fifth estate.

Such groups are not likely to fade away: like the dissenting expert and the food industry public relations machine, the non-governmental *ad hoc* expert committee seems likely to be a continuing component of the food and health debate. Prestigious sponsoring bodies such as the British Medical Association or the Royal College of Physicians are unlikely to renounce their right to produce such reports. As long as they continue, other grand-sounding bodies, such as the London Food Commission or the British Nutrition Foundation, or the National Advisory Committee on Nutrition Education, will produce appropriate counterblasts.

Expert Committees: The Interface of Science and Government

Even if all policy-related decisions were to be concentrated into a few governmental expert committees there would still be grounds for our concern. The expert committee has proved to be extremely flawed in the *way* in which it functions. The most obvious example, which Cannon [9] and others have (in my view quite rightly) criticised, is the secrecy within which the official committees function, and this is one of many areas where the blanket application of the Official Secrets Act, and similar attitudes to the Civil Service, must be reviewed.

But there are other, equally pressing, flaws which led Scrimshaw [14] to write in a retrospective view of his own activities:

It is, of course, well recognised that committees in any discipline are fallible, and some have made monumental blunders using what were regarded as the best minds and information available at the time . . . Overall we have discovered no better system, but in any specific case, the possibility of committee error must be recognised. The error may be no fault of the committee but rather a consequence of inadequate data. However, it may be for a variety of reasons, among them poor selection of members, personality and prestige factors, and failure to identify and evaluate all relevant data. [14]

Specifically in the context of the WHO/FAO Expert Committee on Energy and Protein Requirements [13] he continued:

I must conclude . . . that the committee members, including myself, often acted without sufficient detailed and first hand knowledge of all the relevant literature; that background documents and unpublished data presented at the time of the meeting usually failed to receive sufficient consideration because once the meeting began, no one had the time to study them; and that prior personal positions and biases of individual committee members were not always overcome...

Reviewing personal experience as a participant in dozens of expert, technical and advisory committees over the past 20 years, I am impressed that the most dogmatic and outspoken committee members on any issue may turn out subsequently to have been mistaken on that issue. There have also been occasions when a strong and persistent dissenter has been proved to be right. We need constantly to remind ourselves that neither individuals nor committees are always infallible, and that all scientific issues need to be addressed with some humility. In particular, the democratic approach to scientific truth is a contradiction in terms – the truth may most often be with the majority, but it is not always. The dissenters should be listened to carefully. [15]

Scrimshaw's words echo those of Greenwood, Professor of Vital Statistics in my own institution and chairman of the first UK Ministry of Health Advisory Committee on Nutrition until 1934. He wrote to Hudson, the secretary of the committee:

. . . the democratic method of settling matters of dispute by voting does not seem applicable to scientific questions . . . there is not at present sufficient agreement among those whose experience gives them the right of judgement for it to be possible to advise the Ministry on many of the problems submitted. [Greenwood 1933, cited from reference 12]

Greenwood and Scrimshaw touch on a problem which continues to beset the system. If a government wishes for clear and positive policy advice it must restrict the committee's membership to experts who are likely to agree in their interpretation of evidence. Whereas, if what is required is a review of the current state of knowledge, then the committee must include experts whose interpretations of the evidence will differ.

In my view, this dilemma could be resolved by breaking with the cabal model of expert committees and proceeding further towards Cannon's judicial model. I have argued elsewhere that:

The committees must no longer meet in private, publishing no minutes and basing their cogitations on working papers that, in contradiction to the basic ethos of science, are not available [publicly] for criticism, confirmation or rebuttal. We need to have the process of establishing their membership clear and in the public domain. It must be borne in mind that experts tend to believe passionately in their own theories, and, in that sense, are *least* suited to arrive at a balanced judgement in that field of science.

If only experts are to meet in these committees it must be ensured that all points of view are represented . . . we need them to be so structured that they are not cabals of chums but debating chambers where views are discussed by interested experts, or even scientific courts where an idea is presented by its proponents, and subjected to cross examination by an expert whose job is to expose its flaws, and where the outcome is decided by the impartial jury of competent but disinterested scientists, not experts already wedded to one point of view. [16]

Such proposals have so far attracted only two types of criticism. First that the present system functions so well that they are unnecessary, and second that they are utopian, a description which is intended, I assume, as a simile for incovenient, but which I regard as a compliment. No one has suggested to me that such changes would impair the ability of expert committees to arrive at a scientifically acceptable consensus, appropriate for use in food policy.

Of course, though it might seem self-evident that the function of official expert committees is to arrive at such a consensus, it would be good to remember the point made with regard to the nuclear weapons debate. In the political arena health and human life, like motherhood, is something you do not vote against. Therefore though the state may in effect be setting off health gain against losses in a non-health area, it prefers not to appear to do so. We therefore have a situation where a debate which is in fact about, let us say, the relative implications of food policy for the economy and for health, will be presented as though it is about the quality of the evidence for an effect of food policy on health. Not to put too fine a point on it, there may be advantages to the politician in a committee which can be guaranteed not to reach a decision, for reasons which R. H. S. (Dick) Crossman summed up in his diaries, written at a time when he was Minister of Health and Social Security: "the official machine with its official committees not only reaches administrative conclusions but political conclusions as well" [17]. It is the essentially political nature of their decisions that means that while scientists are being invited to advise "impartially", their sphere of action may be kept constrained by politicians or civil servants.

I do not know how one should deal with this problem, since it touches the central issue of political power, something Whitehall will not wish to relinquish. Indeed, it is not self-evident that scientific advisory committees should somehow be kept pure and aloof from the governments which may implement their views. On the eve of a Labour government and in the now faded white heat of the technological revolution, Crossman argued the converse. Planning he felt:

requires definition of clearly defined targets to which the community's efforts can be directed: and . . . it can only be successfully achieved by the systematic use of scientific methods both in the investigation which precedes selection of the aims, and in plans worked out to achieve them . . . we now need, in peace as well as in war, the constant reinvigoration of our professional administrators in Whitehall from outside. [18]

It is worth noting that Crossman saw this process as needing not sporadic sittings of committees but periods of two to three years of contract work by academics, something which he rightly suggested would undoubtedly improve the vitality of academic research.

In Crossman's view the aloof occasional committee is not a council of perfection but, given the structure of the bureaucratic machine, a recipe for failure. This is the same point made by Lord Snow, in his Godkin Lectures on Science and Government, who suggested that:

to be any real good, the committee has to possess (or take . . .) powers of action. It needs at the least the power of inspection and follow-up. If it does not have those, it will be too far from the reality it is trying to decide about, and too far away from the people who are supposed to carry out the decisions. Advisory committees, if they are confined to pure advice and never get near the point of action, fade away into a kind of accidie. [19]

Snow was writing of the simplest kind of scientific committee which is that involved in the gadgetry of warfare. Indeed his specific model was the Tizard committee which successfully got the British defensive radar. That public health committees are more politically complex is, I hope, by now obvious. Perhaps the wartime functioning of the Ministry of Food committees, the documents of which are now coming into the public domain, will provide clearer guidance on this point of the optimal structures for such expert groups.

In making my criticism of official expert committees, I do not deny what the existing structure has achieved. Committees framing nutrition policy have improved food policy in ways none of us would deny, for example by ensuring the production of low-solute baby foods. They have also introduced policy which has harmed health, as with the wartime over-fortificiation of National Dried Milk, which led to many infant deaths from hypervitaminosis D (idiopathic hypercalcaemia) [23].

Nutritionists are, in my view, too prone to claim great successes for their activities in the policy arena. Although food supply has improved in the last 100 years, much of that change came from the impact of technology rather than food policy. In late Victorian Britain agriculture was in decline while food supply improved, a result of unregulated and unplanned imports from the United States, South America and the Empire (see Chap. 8). In the inter-war period the nutritional aspects of food policy were overwhelmingly concerned with improving vitamin intakes, when the major nutritional problem was underfeeding. Consequently policies were not unequivocal successes. For example, the introduction of school milk, which displaced the feeding of subsidised or free school dinners, reduced the energy and protein value, and increased the cost, of school feeding [12].

The wartime food policy which is often held up as a model for our times, can be criticised, and has yet to be properly evaluated for its health impact. It was undoubtedly an heroic undertaking by patriots in an Homeric situation. Its egalitarianism may well have done much to ensure national unity, its existence may have prevented a decline in the nation's health, but whether it actually altered the *status quo*, as current mythology has it, is open to doubt [23].

I am willing to concede that, on balance, the UK committees over the last 50 years may well have had a beneficial influence on health. That is not the point at issue. The issue is that currently the structure attracts criticism, particularly from a vocal consumerist lobby that wants what Sanders calls food puritanism, draconian changes in the diet, and extensive restrictions on additive use. I do not agree with the consumerists' scientific reasoning, but I recognise their political power, which arises from their popularity and a disillusionment with science and government on the part of the general public.

I also recognise that there is a considerable scientific acceptance of an increased role for diet in the aetiology of degenerative disease, and hence demand for changes in nutrition policy and its incorporation into food policy [24]. All this gives the activities of expert committees in nutrition a high political profile. I do not believe the present system will survive these dual pressures. I would rather it was rationally reformed than overthrown for narrow political reasons.

Food and Nutrition Policy and the Structure of Science

There is one final issue I wish to address. Whatever the reforms in the functioning of the advisory system might be, it is clear that food policy is again firmly on the political agenda, to a degree that rivals, perhaps even surpasses, its pinnacle of importance in World War II. The nature of the political process has undergone some profound changes since then, most notably in the development of a clear consumer lobby that expects stances on issues from professional groups, and will have no truck with closed politics. Such viewpoints will, indeed already do, impinge upon the scientific community, and will result in an increasing demand that scientists adopt consensus or group views about public health topics. At some point this issue will have to be faced by nutritionists as it has already been faced by dietitians with regard to diet, or the medical profession with regard to smoking.

Nutritionists have organised themselves into a society which has adopted the tradition of not holding views on topics. Many of us are comfortable with this, but I doubt that it will last. Some professional body is going to have to take a lead in being a body which purports to represent the consensus amongst nutritional scientists. Personally I have no doubt that a coherent response will come soonest from the medical profession, which within its complex professional structure is quite able to tolerate scientific indecision, clinical certainty and the existence of para-political campaigns, such as the one which the British Medical Association (BMA) is now mounting against smoking. Anyone who reads the BMA book on the subject must be struck not only by the fact that the BMA sees itself in this campaign as one of the pressure groups, but that its tone is firmly wedded to the language of politics.

If the BMA begins to campaign on diet and health, and to argue the need for a new comprehensive food and health policy, nutritionists will have to decide whether they want the policial campaign to be mounted by a body to which most cannot belong, or if not, which body they wish to represent them in the political arena. The nutritionists' ideal of the disinterested group of concerned scientists may not have long to last.

Conclusion

In this discussion I have adopted a philosophy of "it ain't what you do, it's the way that you do it", deliberately shielding my views on what it is I think should be done. However, I have done so because I am satisfied that the scientific debate about causes and prevention is now a vigorous one, which progresses, in a specific sense, continually. The resolution of that debate will come only with better experimental data, not more resumés of the current evidence. But the translation of science into policy involves more than proof, and will proceed without proof. To those who think that "the way that you do it" is irrelevant, I commend the next line of the Fats Waller song: "That's what gets results".

Therefore it is reasonable to ask ourselves whether we are satisfied with the way in which this policy is guided, and with its impact upon us. These are to me the primary questions, and I believe that we need a symposium on these issues before we have yet another one on what should be in that policy.

References

1.   Newton K (1982) The theory of pluralist democracy. In: McGrew AG, Wilson MJ (eds) Decision making, approaches and analysis. Manchester University Press, Manchester
2.   Richardson JJ, Jordan AG (1979) Governing under pressure. Martin Robertson, London
3.   Lindblom CE (1979) Still muddling, not yet through. Publ Admin 39:517–526
4.   Rivers J, Payne PR (1979) Why eating should carry a government health warning. Nature 291:98–99
5.   Cochrane AL (1972) Effectiveness and efficiency. Random reflections on health services. The Nuffield Provincial Hospitals Trust, London
6.   Lord Rothschild (1978) Risk. Listener, 30 November, pp 715–718
7.   Committee on Medical Aspects of Food Policy (1974) Diet and coronary heart disease. DHSS report on health and social subjects 7. HMSO, London
8.   Marmot MG (1986) Epidemiology and the art of the soluble. Lancet I:897–900
9.   Cannon G (1987) The politics of food. Century Hutchinson, London
10. Popper K (1959) The logic of scientific discovery. Hutchinson, London
11. NACNE (1983) A discussion paper on proposals for nutritional guidelines for health education in Britain. Health Education Council, London
12. Petty EC (1987) The impact of the newer knowledge of nutrition: nutrition science and nutrition policy, 1900–1939. PhD thesis, University of London
13. FAO/WHO (1973) Energy and protein requirements. WHO Technical Report Series 522. WHO, Geneva
14. Scrimshaw NS (1976) Shattuck lecture. Strengths and weaknesses of the committee approach. An analysis of past and present recommended dietary allowances for protein in health and disease, part 1. N Engl J Med 294:136–143
15. Scrimshaw NS (1976) Shattuck Lecture. Strengths and weaknesses of the committee approach. An analysis of past and present recommended dietary allowances for protein in health and disease, part 2. N Engl J Med 294:198–203
16. Rivers J (1986) A long-handled spoon. Nutr News Notes 13:1–3
17. Crossman RHS (1977) The diaries of a cabinet minister, volume 3. Secretary of state for social services, 1968–1970. Hamish Hamilton and Jonathan Cape, London
18. Crossman RHS (1964) Scientists in Whitehall. Encounter 13(1):3–10
19. Snow CP (1961) Science and government. Oxford University Press, London, p 75
20. Payne P, Thomson A (1979) Food health: individual choice and collective responsibility. J R Soc Health, 185–189
21. Marshall E (1985) The Academy kills a nutrition report. Science 230:420–421
22. Marshall E (1986) Diet advice, with a grain of salt and a large helping of pepper. Science 231:537–539
23. Rivers JPW (1979) The profession of nutrition – an historical perspective. Proc Nutr Soc 38: 255–231
24. Anonymous (1986) Britain needs a food and health policy: the government must face its duty. Lancet II:434–436 (editorial)

Commentary

Note by Southgate on RDAs: Recommended Daily Allowances should be regarded as guidelines for those constructing or evaluating diets.

They encapsulate the need to cover the minimum amounts of nutrients to prevent deficiency disease, plus arbitrary safety factors and limits to prevent excessive intakes. However, these are not their sole uses, nor do they represent the physiological requirements for nutrients.

The major problems are firstly that their presentation as numerical values for guidance leads to the numbers being used inappropriately without recognition of the limited precision of the numerical values; and secondly that they are used for individuals, whereas they can only provide guidance for groups.

Note by Sanders on RDAs: It may be unwise to stipulate recommended daily intakes for those nutrients the requirements for which are uncertain, and when deficiency disease is unknown.

Sanders: This paper is an interesting discourse on the philosophy behind having a food and nutrition policy. Yet I was disappointed because it did not discuss current policies and their basis in sufficient detail. We clearly do have a policy in the United Kingdom. I think that what many of the protagonists mean when they say we do not have a food and nutrition policy is that their personal views on the relationship between diet and disease are not accepted by the Establishment. There obviously is a need to define more clearly what the policy objectives should be in both health and socioeconomic terms. It is difficult in any policy area to quantify factors numerically as proposed by Joy and Payne. However, there are surely certain areas where there is a consensus on food and nutrition policy: for example the need to protect the consumer from acute damage to his or her health and from fraud. Successive governments have had policies with regard to how infants and children should be fed.

The "global strategy" of advocating one set of dietary guidelines for the whole population has obvious limitations because the needs for food change throughout life. The relative risks of a change in diet need to be carefully assessed. Take for example the case for decreasing sugar intakes. On the one hand, the replacement of sugar by artificial sweeteners may decrease the risk of dental caries and may help decrease energy intakes, but on the other hand sweeteners may carry with them their own specific risks. The argument of the food puritan is that you should not consume either: if a food is enjoyable then it cannot be good for you. The pleasure derived from eating food is another factor that needs to taken into account in any policy.

The mechanism by which government reaches decisions concerning food and nutrition policy is bewildering to many nutritionists. For example, in the COMA report on cardiovascular disease, a decision was made to include *trans* fatty acids with saturated fatty acids for the labelling recommendations. This recommendation broke new ground, but the basis for it was not explained nor referenced in the report. Subsequently published reports by the British Nutrition Foundation Task Force on *trans* fatty acids and by the Federation of American Societies for Experimental Biology were unable to show a link between the consumption of *trans* fatty acids and arterial disease. The Department of Health and Social Security (DHSS) refused to explain why *trans* fatty acids were being included with saturated fatty acids by invoking the Official Secrets Act. The DHSS has refused to change its view on this issue and has recently reaffirmed its intention to require manufacturers to include *trans* fatty acids with saturated fatty acids in nutritional labelling. While there may be some areas where secrecy is essential for the proper working of government, for example on matters of defence, it is absurd that the British diet, feared throughout the world, is a state secret.

This paper might have considered the implications of the current guidelines and what they might achieve in terms of disease reduction and what the economic implications might be. Another issue is whether we should express intakes of nutrients on an energy basis or as absolute intakes.

Durnin: I think that Sanders' suggestion that the DHSS "refused to explain . . . by invoking the Official Secrets Act" is probably based on misunderstanding. It is certainly quite at variance with my own experience on several government advisory bodies on "nutrition". After a report has been published, or made public, I should be very surprised to think that the DHSS would not be prepared either to explain matters to the best of their ability, or to refer the questioner to the appropriate professional adviser, usually the chairman of the relevant group. *Before* the report has been properly discussed and agreed by the expert committee, it would obviously be inappropriate for the DHSS to give detailed explanations, which, in a matter involving much controversy, could easily be at variance with the views of some members of the committee.

Thomas: The difference between a food policy and a nutrition policy has been spelt out by Whitehead [1]:

Essentially a food policy makes certain that people have access to safe, wholesome food of the type they like to eat, in sufficient amounts to meet demands; a nutrition policy, on the other hand, is primarily concerned with the nutrient quality of the diet in terms of the optimisation of human health. In practice of course, the difference is not clear cut, but it is important to realise that the terms are not synonymous.

Consequently, while it is possible to have a food policy as defined above where nutrition and health considerations have a fairly low priority, it is impossible to have a nutrition policy without those elements of agricultural and economic planning which traditionally form the planks of a food policy.

It is this difference in emphasis which has underpinned calls in recent years for a national nutrition policy, resulting in an area for debate which is arguably much wider than Rivers would have us believe. A central question remains: is there a need for a food policy to be replaced by a nutrition policy?

Not that the issue is new. In its report of 1937 the League of Nations [2] identified two distinct, though mutually dependent aims for any successful nutrition policy. Its primary concern should be with consumption, i.e. with bringing the foods essential for health and physical development within the reach of all sections of the community. But in addition a nutrition policy must consider supply. It must take into account the problems surrounding the adaptation of agriculture and possibly of commerce to changes in demand and of increasing supply as demand expands.

As Nichola Bull [3] has pointed out, "the history of nutrition policy appears rather like a wheel, turning, but advancing little, of which we only see one arc as it appears periodically". In order to make some progress, clarification or just what sort of policy (with what aims) was under discussion, would have helped in the consideration of how such policy should be developed. It would have put Rivers' discussion of "conflict between outcomes" into a context where a deeper analysis was possible, and it clearly has implications for discussion of costs and benefits.

Many valuable points are raised in the discussion of experts and committees, particularly the need to avoid the "herd instinct", which, as Sir William Beveridge pointed out, "gives widely held beliefs a spurious validity irrespective of whether or not they are founded on any real evidence" [4]. One important aspect which might have benefited from some comment relates to the interdisciplinary nature of advice required in framing a coherent policy. Marks [5] and many other authors have highlighted the way in which fragmentation of responsibility between different government departments results in a lack of integrated policy. An example of this was clearly identified by the Royal Commission on Environmental Pollution [6] when considering the involvement of the Ministry of Agriculture, Fisheries and Food and the Department of the Environment in pollution issues. Rivers' thoughts on possible advice structures which might avoid similar lacunae in relation to nutrition/health/agriculture issues would be most interesting, and would inevitably raise questions about the ability of scientists with different specialities to communicate and cooperate with each other. The latter point is of some relevance to Rivers' final comments on food and nutrition policy and the structure of science. I was rather perplexed, though, by the reference to dietitians as a group which had faced and come to terms with the demand to adopt a consensus view on diet, apparently in contrast to nutritionists. Since dietetics is the "application of the science of nutrition in the feeding of people in sickness and health", it is hard to see how dietitians could escape the same dilemmas as nutritionists.

References

1. Whitehead RG (1978) Food policy and health. The E. F. Armstrong memorial lecture. J R Soc Arts 126: 552–563
2. League of Nations (1937) Mixed committee on the relation of nutrition to health, agriculture and economic policy.
3. Bull L (1978) The nutritionist's role in UK food policy 1937–77. MSc thesis, Faculty of medicine, University of London
4. Beveridge W (1950) The art of scientific investigation. Heinemann, London
5. Marks L (1984) Public health and agricultural practice. Food Policy 9: 131–138
6. Royal Commission on Environmental Pollution (1979) Seventh report: agriculture and pollution. HMSO, London

Southgate: This paper addresses some extremely fundamental issues regarding the formulation of any governmental policy, and raises many more questions than it attempts to answer. While it is strictly true that considered inaction can be an expression of policy, this only applies when inaction is a considered response. Inaction because of the inertia of the system and possibly because of the desire to retain the *status quo* is a conservative policy. However, inaction because the evidence is conflicting or partial and because of reluctance to define or accept any standard of proof is not policy.

The matter of standards of proof required to demonstrate that diet is related to health or that changes would benefit health is an important one. Surely we should proceed from the hypothesis that diet and health are related and therefore that a change in diet is associated with a change in health? Replacing "health" by disease incidence produces a relationship that can be analysed quantitatively. Such a hypothesis can be tested formally in a Popperian sense by experimental essays at falsification. On this basis one would have evidence that might be judged on the basis of probability. Another factor that needs to be considered is the evidence of harm. Here, as is pointed out, harm may arise at a distance. Coronary heart disease death rates may fall, while depressed standards of living in the dairy industry may produce more suicides, broken homes or malnutrition for example. Once again input/benefit relationships are undefinable.

Does this mean that we need to accept inaction as a policy because we really cannot weigh the pros and cons, or should we discuss how we should judge them? Can we proceed on the basis that no harm to those consuming the diet is likely, but some benefits are probable?

One aspect of food policy where the government is active is in the support of food production. It would be useful to debate whether this support runs counter to public health issues. It could be argued that the policies for food production should be driven by requirements for food and that an integrated food and nutrition policy would in the longer-term benefit both producer and consumer.

Dobbing: The Editor may not be supposed to write Commentaries, but, as was no doubt intended by the author, this paper is so provocative and interesting that he will pick out a few points.

As a scientist I do not always find it difficult to imagine "an objective way of justifying a price paid by the many in terms of benefit felt by the few". What about insurance? Health insurance? I think I can justify the price scientifically, as well as its moral implications.

We do *not* "tolerate a considerable mortality on the roads so that some may have the freedom to drive". We complain about the mortality and try to reduce or abolish it. This is a "road policy"! A bad example. As is the example of "siting of traffic lights where reduced accident risk is weighed against impact on traffic flow". I do not think this happens as starkly as is suggested. Analogies can be *faux amis*!

When talking about the criteria of proof which cannot be met in the sense of those required in "internal science", I think Rivers is confusing the criteria of scientific proof with those which would only have to be *sufficiently* convincing for the formulation of policy. It sounds as though his "strict scientific criteria", and Marmot's "lust for absolute proof" are being set up as skittles in order to knock them down. Medical doctors, in the interest of action, are constantly formulating policy towards their patients on the basis of *sufficiently* convincing evidence, *faute de mieux*, and there is no reason why nutritionists should not do likewise if they want action. Indeed they are likely to be more honest than doctors about the degree of uncertainty.

I cannot accept Rivers' defence of PR activities, and we do not "just have to live with them". There are ways out, such as the long-term education and vigilance of media reporters, which could be part of a badly needed training. Even our fellow citizens might be taught (at school?) to spot the motives behind the reporting of "news" of all kinds, and the widespread deception behind almost every item on the "Today" programme on Radio 4. That, however, would need a new generation of teachers. This has been done successfully with medical students of clinical pharmacology in relation to pharmaceutical advertising to the profession, and if medical students can learn, then anyone can.

Rivers criticises "sponsoring bodies like the Royal College of Physicians, the British Nutrition Foundation or the Health Education Council". I do not think he should mix up two theoretically altruistic organisations with an overt mouthpiece for the food industry, of which I am not, for that reason, a critic. If he is saying that the common membership of all three committees is dishonest, we should investigate and offer some evidence.

The hold of the vitamin lobby on the Campaign against Mulnutrition may simply have been due to our having fallen, in 1930, for what nutritionists themselves felt at the time was part of the science of nutrition. Cathcart may well have been visionary, but in as much as he was expressing a belief rather than evidence, he may have been for that reason ignored.

Durnin: Although I am sure Rivers would use my following statement to support his own argument, I found little relevance of many of the things he suggests to my own experiences on government advisory committees. He sometimes seems to me to show a complete ignorance of how such committees work and are chosen.

Curzon: Rivers quite rightly makes the point that governmental food policy is very old, dating back to 1266. However, have not nearly all these previous laws been dealing not with food policy *per se* but rather with trade and fraud? I am sure that the legislators of 1266, and those following, were concerned to protect the public from exploitation and *bad* food rather than any idea of healthful eating. What is being advocated is the concept of a food policy as a possible dictation of the type and quality of foods to be used. The question then is whether government should be involved in this at all.

While this issue is addressed by Rivers, the paper should perhaps include a comment on the basic political philosophy as to whether individuals should be left to decide for themselves whether to eat healthy food or not. Coupled with this is the issue of freedom of choice, which in this instance is the freedom of individuals to choose foods for themselves. This is touched upon in terms of whether there should be the freedom to drink and drive. On the question of food, does an individual have the right to eat whatever he pleases even though to do so does not, by and large, affect others?

Naismith: Rivers, it seems to me, has interpreted his brief in too limited a way. His article is concerned largely with the nature of advisory committees (like COMA) and the constraints imposed by politicians and civil servants, and by the reluctance of scientists themselves to compromise on matters of scientific proof. The need for a new basis for formulating government policy is well argued, but the case is over-stated. Government committees like COMA, in dealing with the relationships between diet and health, acknowledge that their recommendations are based on the best scientific opinion currently available. To give one example that illustrates this point: in the COMA report on *Diet and Coronary Heart Disease* published in 1974 an "excess of dietary cholesterol" was listed as a dietary characteristic to be considered as a risk factor for ischaemic heart disease. Ten years and many publications later, in *Diet and Cardiovascular Disease*, it is stated: "evidence for an influence of this level of intake [the current intake] on blood cholesterol is inconclusive", and no specific recommendation is made. In the meantime those who had adjusted their intake of cholesterol in response to government intervention had experienced no harm; this is one of the reassuring things about recommendations on nutritional matters.

In some instances a recommendation not to increase one's intake further (current COMA views on salt and sugar) is misinterpreted as inactivity, but is in fact a true reflection of the state of the scientific evidence (see papers by MacGregor and Durnin). Their apparent timidity, in comparison with the recommendations of other bodies, is to be commended. A radical change in dietary habits is a great deal more complicated, particularly for the social groups in which the so-called diseases of afflu-ence are most prevalent, than a change of prescription.

Although government and industry are attacked with equal vigour by writers such as Cannon, to whom Rivers refers, it is worth noting that the spectacular improve-ment in one aspect of the public malaise, dental caries, has come about by the pro-motion of the prophylactic use of fluoride by the drug industry, encouraged by altruistic dentists. I suspect that the recommendations of both NACNE and the BMA reports on sucrose consumption will have an effect on the incidence of caries that is somewhat less than spectacular.

The dilemma facing a government bent on a policy of mass diet therapy will become apparent to any reader of this book: that all of the clinical conditions dis-cussed – coronary heart disease, obesity, diabetes, hypertension and dental caries – have an important genetic component. The choice is between identifying those pre-disposed to the condition and those who will respond to diet modification (even more difficult), which would be prohibitively expensive, or advocating changes for the entire population, which costs practically nothing. The costs and benefits have clearly been weighed.

How Rivers might have interpreted his title more liberally is by considering whether the general public responds to exhortations from panels of experts, and if the evidence suggests that they do not, then at whom should government policy be directed?

References

DHSS (1974) Diet and coronary heart disease. Report on health and social subjects 7. HMSO, London
DHSS (1984) Diet and cardiovascular disease. Report on health and social subjects 28. HMSO, London

Subject Index